PROMOTION OF MENTAL HEALTH
VOLUME 7, 2000

Promotion of Mental Health
Volume 7, 2000

Edited by

MICHAEL C. MURRAY
COLIN A. REED
The Clifford Beers Foundation

Routledge
Taylor & Francis Group

LONDON AND NEW YORK

First published 2001 by Ashgate Publishing

Reissued 2018 by Routledge
2 Park Square, Milton Park, Abingdon, Oxon OX14 4RN
711 Third Avenue, New York, NY 10017, USA

Routledge is an imprint of the Taylor & Francis Group, an informa business

Notice:
Product or corporate names may be trademarks or registered trademarks, and are used only for identification and explanation without intent to infringe.

Publisher's Note
The publisher has gone to great lengths to ensure the quality of this reprint but points out that some imperfections in the original copies may be apparent.

Disclaimer
The publisher has made every effort to trace copyright holders and welcomes correspondence from those they have been unable to contact.

A Library of Congress record exists under LC control number: 92010714

ISBN 13: 978-1-138-72708-3 (hbk)
ISBN 13: 978-1-138-72706-9 (pbk)
ISBN 13: 978-1-315-19101-0 (ebk)

Contents

Note: a selection of the above papers have been included in a conference issue of The International Journal of Mental Health Promotion.

List of Contributors

Barry, Margaret M. National University of Ireland, Galway
Billington, D.R. Health Organization, Geneva
Birch, Mike. Falmouth College of Art
Booth, Adrian. South Australian Health Commission
Brown, Jane. University of Glasgow
Brugha, T.S. University of Leicester
Burford, Angela. South Australian Health Commission
Burtney, Elizabeth. Health Education Board for Scotland
Dalgard, Odd Steffen. National Institute for Public Health, Oslo
Doherty, Ann. National University of Ireland, Galway
Dwivedi, Kedar Nath. Child and Family Consultation Service, Northampton
Friedli, Lynne. Health Education Board, London
Frisanco, Renato. Department of Mental Health (DSM), Rome E
Gilleard, Chris. MSW Mental Health Promotion Alliance, London
Grispini, Alessandro. Department of Mental Health (DSM), Rome E
Hayes, Claire. National University of Ireland, Maynooth
Herron, Sandy. University of Nottingham
Keddie, Ken. Arbroath, Scotland
Killoran-Ross, Michael. Ayrshire and Arran Health Board
Kinmond, Kathryn. University of Central Enngland
Kok, Gerjo. University of Maastricht
Lancaster, Rebecca J. Institute of Occupational Medicine
Lobo, Ros. MSW Mental Health Promotion Alliance, London
Macdonald, Glenn. University of Central England
Mauthner, Natasha. University of Edinburgh
Mortimer, Rebecca. University of Nottingham
Murphy, Christine. University of Liverpool
Murray, Michael C. The Clifford Beers Foundation
O'Doherty, Elaine. Homefirst Community Trust, Ballymena
Oppedal, Brit. National Institute for Public Health, Oslo
Piccione, Renato. Department of Mental Health (DSM), Rome E
Stacey, Kathleen. Flinders University, Australia
Walsh, Graeme. Lanarkshire Health Board
Wheatley, Sandra L. University of Leicester

Acknowledgements

My first venture into mental health, or perhaps at that time more appropriate to say mental illness, was when I was invited to manage a psychiatric hospital. I hasten to add the invitation came not on the basis of my knowledge of mental health but because, like many other similar institutions, the hospital was ready for an enquiry and I had experience of working in a hostile industrial relations climate.

Even allowing for the fact that I knew very little about mental health it was patently clear that the service we provided was inhumane, expensive and ineffective. Unfortunately the patients had little say in the matter.

Quickly realising there must be a more appropriate way to provide care I sought advice and counsel from colleagues in a series of seminars and at conferences where I learnt from others and on occasions perhaps others learned from me. This sharing of knowledge was of mutual benefit and for those working within a climate of scarce resources helped overcome the wasteful practice of trying to "re-invent the wheel."

When the opportunity arose we tried to put some of the advice received into practice and commissioned a mental health promotion unit. Although we "only had a candle" to light the way and even as we often stumbled in the dark, with help and encouragement from others a clearer path began to emerge.

One of the fruits of our collaboration with others in a similar position was the European Conference on the Promotion of Mental Health which over the years has provided a vehicle for the exchange of knowledge and experiences and for the establishment of networks for practitioners from across national and cultural barriers. This is the seventh volume in the Promotion of Mental Health series which will, I hope, further disseminate the lessons we have learned and the experiences we shared at the European Conferences.

In Volume Seven we have endeavoured to build upon the framework developed by Dr Dennis Trent; the one person who can rightly take credit for the reporting of the Conference proceedings throughout the 1990s. We have sought to bring together the ideas and practices of a diverse group of people bound together with the common aim of securing the rightful place of mental health promotion on the political, health and social and economic agenda. I hope we have managed to maintain Dr Trent's tradition.

It is incumbent upon me to thank all those who have made Volume 7, in the series. It is not possible to include everyone but I could not fail to thank Colin Reed. It is because of Colin that this publication became a reality. Through his abilities and talents and not a little hard work Colin got us here.

Finally to all who contributed my thanks. Without you there would be no collection of ideas to take forward and promote mental health.

M. C. Murray

1 Mental Health Promotion in a Rural Context: Research and Realities from a Community-based Initiative in Northern Ireland

MARGARET M. BARRY, ELAINE O' DOHERTY AND ANN DOHERTY

Abstract

This paper describes the development of mental health promotion strategies for rural communities in a Northern Ireland setting. The initial phase of a community-based project targeting depression and suicide is examined. The paper brings together practitioner and research perspectives on an analysis of the factors that made this initiative possible and facilitated its development to date. This includes the process of establishing policy support for the initiative, consultation with stakeholder groups, and the carrying out of a needs assessment study. The paper is written in two sections. Section one describes the process and practical experience of planning and implementing the initial phase of the project. It details the background factors which helped to resolve the difficulties and challenges encountered in developing mental health promotion practice in a community health and social services trust setting. Section two reports on the community needs assessment study. The research approach adopted in the needs assessment is outlined and the implications of the findings from a community study on perceptions and beliefs concerning mental health issues are discussed.

Background to the Project

Northern Ireland's Regional Strategy for Health and Wellbeing 1997-2002 (DHSS, 1996) has identified the need for a strategy for mental health promotion for Northern Ireland. This is a challenge that various agencies are currently working to meet. Homefirst is a community trust serving a largely rural population (305,000) in Northern Ireland. In line with recent developments, the Trust has sought to develop mental health promotion strategies to meet the needs of the population it serves.

The initiative reported here arose from a community development project known as the Rural Community Development and Health (RCDH) project, which was a three year pilot project set up to explore community development and health approaches in a rural setting (HCT, 1998). This project highlighted the growing problems encountered by people living in rural areas. These include social isolation, unemployment, poor housing, lack of public transport, and lack of public amenities. In addition, recent years have brought a succession of farming crises that have led to financial stresses and further job losses. Against this background there is a steadily rising incidence of depression and suicide (Foster, Gillespie and McClelland, 1997). Focus group research conducted in the Republic of Ireland (Hope et al., 1998) has also highlighted the growing concern among members of the farming community about the rising rates of suicide and depression.

The current project was developed in order to devise innovative and effective strategies for delivering mental health promotion programmes to rural communities. The community-based project is modelled on an existing study designed to promote health and wellbeing in rural communities in the Republic of Ireland (Barry, Hope, Kelleher and Sixsmith, 1998). This paper focuses on stage one of the project which entails the process of engaging the community and local professional groups, undertaking a community needs assessment and developing a plan of action for the intervention phase. The next section traces the project's development in terms of the policy background and the practical experience to date of planning and implementation in a small rural community in mid-Ulster.

Section One: The Process of Project Initiation and Development

Throughout the initiation phase comprehensive documentation was maintained, of all steps taken and all contacts made, as part of monitoring the process of developing the project. While it is too soon to draw conclusions about effective approaches for project replication, it is possible at this stage to identify some of the elements that have contributed to moving mental health promotion forward at a strategic and operational level in the Trust.

A key factor is the infrastructure of health promotion within the Trust. As recommended by the 1995 Review of Health Promotion in Northern Ireland (Neuberger, 1995), Homefirst adopted a range of measures aimed at achieving better integration of health promotion into the Trust. For mental health promotion this means liaising regularly with the Mental Health Senior Management Team to discuss initiatives being undertaken, and explore ways of moving towards a strategy for mental health promotion for the Trust. Many of the difficulties so often encountered in promoting mental health, such as those arising from different conceptualisations and interpretations of mental health, highlighted by MacDonald and O'Hara (1998), have been reduced by the structural arrangements developed within the Trust.

An important element in moving mental health promotion forward strategically in the Trust was the decision by the Senior Management Health Team sub-group to adopt a local community-based initiative as a flagship project. In this way the development of mental health promotion practice is promoted at a concrete project level rather than solely at the more abstract level of a strategy document. This is an approach supported by Secker (1998) which would seem to merit further investigation.

This project started after links were established between the Rural Community Development and Health Project and the Centre for Health Promotion Studies, National University of Ireland, Galway (NUI, Galway) which was undertaking a major health promotion initiative with agri-workers. The Trust's Senior Mental Health Team facilitated the RCDH project to engage with the researchers in developing a similar initiative in a matched location in Homefirst's area. Senior management support has given the project priority status, thus ensuring support and co-operation from local health and social care staff.

A further factor was the intersectoral nature of the project. Gillies (1998) demonstrates that alliance or partnership initiatives do work in tackling the broader determinants of health. The RCDH project was carried out by a partnership of community, voluntary and statutory sector organisations, including Homefirst Community Trust. Undoubtedly the partnership of the organisations and agencies prepared to support this project has enhanced the status and credibility of mental health promotion, assisting the process of reorienting the health services.

Resourcing is a factor crucial to the success of any initiative and this project is no exception. The fairly long term funding (i.e. three years) for the

RCDH project facilitated the building of social capital (Gillies, 1998) in the form of a supportive infrastructure of networks and groups. Networks established through the RCDH project provided immediate access to representatives of the local community and key voluntary and statutory agencies. This existing infrastructure was a key element in progressing the current project.

The community development principles of consultation, participation, communication and sustainability which were purposely incorporated into practice, contributed greatly to the level of local support for the project. A research assistant from the local University of Ulster, Jordanstown (UUJ) was employed to help with local consultation, data collection, informing the local community and preparing a report on the RCDH project. A Project Steering Group comprising representatives from the community, health and social care staff, farming organisations and the voluntary sector was established.

Perhaps, most importantly, the research-based approach adopted in the project ensures that programme development and implementation will be built on a sound empirical base. The needs assessment study focusing on current perceptions and attitudes in the community helps to ensure that the programmes developed will be both meaningful and relevant to community members. In addition, the process and outcome evaluation will help inform both policy and practice in this developing area.

Section Two: The Needs Assessment Study - Community Perceptions and Beliefs Concerning Mental Health Issues

A research framework to support the development and implementation of the mental health promotion project was developed by the Centre for Health Promotion Studies (NUI, Galway). The Centre was already undertaking a research-based health promotion in four rural communities in the Republic of Ireland. A small rural community in mid-Ulster, similar in size and profile to that of the rural communities participating in the larger study across the border (i.e. less than 2,000 population), was selected for participation in the study. The research methodology was adapted from the larger study (Barry, Hope, Kelleher and Sixsmith, 1998) in order to allow comparison across the different settings.

The needs assessment study consists of a cross-sectional survey of the attitudes, beliefs and practices of rural people in relation to mental health issues, with a particular focus on depression and suicide. The aim of the study is to inform the development of appropriate interventions and also to provide

4

baseline data against which to measure the success of the intervention strategies. The exploration of community beliefs is also intended to ground the mental health promotion programme in the values and beliefs of the local community and to facilitate community involvement at the early stages of programme development. This approach embraces the implicit theories and views held by community members in order to build the project on the social meanings and understandings of mental health current in the community (Barry, 1998). To this end a cross-sectional survey was carried out in the Autumn of 1997. A summary of the findings of this study will now be presented. Full details of the study are reported in Doherty, Barry and Sixsmith (1998).

Method

Sample

The sample point for the survey was taken as the village centre and interviewers covered an area of a radius of five miles from this point. Households were randomly selected by the researchers calling to every second house in the village area and every house in the open countryside. Quota sampling procedures were used, stratifying according to age and sex. The response rate was 69% and a total of 242 people were surveyed. The characteristics of this sample can be summarised as follows: 43% male, 52% under 40 years of age; 21% had attained a primary standard of education only, with 46% secondary level and 33% third-level. The sample was equally divided between manual and nonmanual occupations and only 10% were categorised as having had a high level of previous contact with mental health problems.

Measures

The main survey technique was an interviewer-administered questionnaire which explored;

   (i)   levels of awareness and knowledge of depression and suicide;
   (ii) current practices and attitudes concerning mental health matters;
   (iii) perceived barriers and benefits of service up-take;
   (iv) perceived confidence in dealing with mental health issues;

(v) stigma;

(vi) sources of information and influences on personal views and beliefs.

One-third of the respondents (N=88) were also questioned using a vignette portraying a person displaying signs of depression and suicidal ideation. The vignette, a short, hypothetical case description written in non-technical language, devised by Barry (1994), was used in order to obtain data of a more qualitative nature concerning the perception and interpretation of depression.

Results

Questionnaire findings Levels of awareness were generally high in the community with 81 % of respondents aware of the rise in the suicide rate in Northern Ireland in the last decade. Some 53% of respondents were concerned about levels of both rural suicide and depression, and 43% reported concern in relation to access to mental health services in rural areas. Of the respondents, men (F = 7.06, p<.01) and those under 40 years of age (F= 13.1, p<.01) were the groups least concerned about levels of suicide in rural areas. The same pattern was found in relation to concern about depression.

With regard to advising someone with depression, 35% of the respondents recommended seeking help from a GP, with 24% also advising nonprofessional support, e.g. from a close friend or family member. Of the remaining responses, 10% endorsed the 'pull yourself together' option and 8% recommended seeing a psychiatrist, 5% recommended the Samaritans and 6% a member of the clergy. Almost half the respondents (46%) said that they would find it difficult to advise someone who was depressed, and 68% reported little confidence in their own ability to advise someone who was suicidal.

In relation to attitudes to services, 59% of respondents felt that going to the GP would be an effective action if depressed. The psychiatrist was endorsed by 67% of respondents. In general, the GP was the professional that people would have the least hesitation in consulting if depressed (72% would not hesitate), followed by the psychiatrist (55%), the psychologist (53%) and the Samaritans (42%). Men was significantly less likely than women to believe in the effectiveness of the GP (F=6.25, p<.05) for treating depression. Again, the under-40 age group was most hesitant about consulting a GP and was also significantly less likely to seek help from a psychiatrist (F = 8.48, p<.01).

Open-ended questions concerning barriers to seeking help revealed that social stigma was the most frequently cited barrier (35%). Respondents also referred to reluctance to disclose their problems (22%) and distrust of the services (7%). Non-recognition of the need for help (3%) and lack of knowledge of where to go for help (2%) were also cited. Analysis of the demographic variables revealed that younger respondents were more likely to cite 'social stigma' as a barrier to help seeking ($x^2=15.01$, $p<.01$).

Further exploring perceptions of the stigma attached to mental health problems revealed that the majority of respondents would not talk openly about someone close to them receiving treatment for depression. Only 27% reported that they would talk openly, 15% would keep it hidden and 38% would talk only to close friends. These figures are much lower than those reported by Sogaard and Fonnebo (1995) in a recent Norwegian Mental Health Survey where 66.6% declared that they would talk openly about the matter. Concerning disclosing personal matters with others, just over half the respondents (57%) reported that they had discussed their 'joys and sorrows' with members of their families in the last month. Slightly fewer (53%) had discussed the same matters with members outside their families. Women ($x^2=11.13$, $p<.01$) and those with third-level education ($x^2= 8.4$, $p <.05$) were significantly more likely to talk about their joys and sorrows with others.

Concerning sources of influence on beliefs about mental health matters, the GP and members of one's family and friends were the most commonly named influential sources. Most respondents expressed the view that leaflets, television, other people, and talks locally would be the best ways of delivering messages on mental health to them. In this rural community local media (radio and newspapers) were named more frequently than national media.

Vignette study findings In response to the vignette case, 67% of respondents recognised the symptoms of depression as portrayed by the vignette actor. Women were significantly more likely than men to recognise the vignette actor's problem as depression ($x^2=5.67$, $p<.05$). There was general recognition (84%) that the problem was a serious one.

In terms of causal explanations, social isolation (35%) and having a negative outlook on life (16%) were referred to most frequently as causes of the vignette actor's problems. The most popular advice offered to the vignette actor (by 65% of respondents) was to use self-help tactics such as 'get out and meet people'. Over one-third of responses advised consulting the GP, and 24% advised seeking non-professional support form friends and family. Most respondents (66%) expressed the view that the vignette actor had a good chance of recovering and 48% felt that s/he would be received positively by the community.

Discussion

The findings from the vignette and the questionnaire reveal the levels of awareness, stigma and attitudes among members of this rural community and point to a number of issues that need to be addressed in the interventions. While general levels of knowledge and concern in relation to depression and suicide are high, they were lowest among those conceivably at highest risk, i.e. males and the younger age groups. There also appeared to be low awareness of the risk of suicide linked to depression. Respondents in this study failed to make a connection between suicide and depression, even when overtly referenced in the vignette.

Symptom recognition and help-seeking emerge as particular issues for younger adults and males. The study found that men were less likely than women to recognise the symptoms of depression or to perceive the problem to be serious. Men also expressed lower levels of concern in relation to depression and suicide and were also more optimistic about recovery prospects. These factors may be indicative of a lack of awareness on the part of men as to the nature and severity of depression. Likewise, men and the under 40 age group showed a greater reluctance to consult a professional about mental health problems.

There was a general lack of confidence among respondents in dealing with depression and suicide in others or advising them about where to go for help, even when the symptoms are recognised. With regard to services, belief in the efficacy of professional services was generally high. However, males and the under 40 age group were less willing to consult the services and was also less likely to believe in their effectiveness.

Concerning disclosure and confiding in others, there appeared to be a general reluctance to share one's worries and joys with others. This was particularly so among males. The value of interpersonal communication and the use of informal sources of support, such as family and peers, needs to be highlighted for rural males.

The issue of stigma and negative attitudes at the community level need to be addressed, particularly the implications for the younger age group. Social stigma emerged as potentially the biggest barrier to seeking outside help for depression among the under- 40 age group. The family and the G.P. were the most frequently named influential source on mental health matters. Interventions should capitalise on the 'close to home' nature of influences and also take into account the potentially important role of the family doctor.

The findings point to the need for programmes for men and younger adults in rural areas concerning issues of depression and suicide. The importance of local influences in the rural context highlight the need for a strong community-based focus to underpin the development of programmes addressing the needs of the different target groups. The intervention should also seek to address the role of more informal support networks within the community such as family and peers as well as inter-agency programmes involving voluntary and statutory agencies and support groups.

Dissemination of Findings

In order to formulate a plan of action for the intervention phase the findings from the needs assessment study were reported back to the local community and health and social care staff. This took the form of a series of conferences and public meetings. A draft report on the survey's findings was prepared. Consultation meetings included presentations, workshops and discussion groups were held on issues arising from the survey findings. Following this local consultation, the survey report and recommendations were published. A summary report was sent to everyone who attended the conference and to all those involved in the project.

Conclusions

In summary, the steps towards the success of the project to date include: the commitment of the Trust's Health Promotion Department to a research based approach to mental health promotion; the strategy of integration into the Trust adopted by the Health Promotion Department; the linking up with highly reputable, experienced partners; the securing of Trust senior management support and commitment; and the adoption of a community based approach in the project. Among the difficulties to be tackled were uncertainty and mistrust among health and social services staff of the concept of mental health promotion; the need to establish effective communication channels with the local community and local health and social services staff.

The needs assessment study clearly points to the need to reach men and younger adults in order to raise awareness and confidence in relation to mental health issues and to reduce levels of stigma. Given the rural context, this needs to be embedded within a community-wide initiative in order to create a supportive climate for planned interventions. The lessons learned from phase one of the project are now being applied in the next phase of the programme which entails developing, implementing and evaluating programmes in the rural community setting.

References

Barry, M. M. (1994) 'Community perceptions of mental disorder: an Irish perspective', *The Irish Journal of Psychology*, 15, (2&3), pp. 418-441.

Barry, M. M. (1998) 'The role of lay beliefs and perceptions in the development of mental health promotion strategies', in M. K. Ross and C. Stark (eds) *Promoting Mental Health*, Ayr Organising Committee of the Ayrshire International Mental Health Promotion Conference, 1997.

Barry, M. M., Hope, A., Kelleher, C. C. and Sixsmith, J. (1998) 'Evaluation of a community-based mental health promotion programme among rural residents', *Unpublished paper*, Centre for Health Promotion Studies, National University of Ireland, Galway.

DHSS (1995) *Health Promotion Arrangements in Northern Ireland*, Report of a review group under the chairmanship of Rabbi Julia Neuberger, DHSS.

DHSS (1996) *Health and Wellbeing: Into the Millennium. Regional Strategy for Health and Social Wellbeing 1997-2002*, HMSO, Belfast.

Doherty, A., Barry, M. M. and Sixsmith, J. (1998) *Health and Social Wellbeing in a Rural Community: Community Perceptions and Beliefs Concerning Mental Health Issues*, Centre for Health Promotion Studies, National University of Ireland, Galway.

Foster, T., Gillespie, K. and McClelland, R. (1997) 'Mental Disorders and Suicide in Northern Ireland', *British Journal of Psychiatry*, 170, pp. 447-452.

Gillies, P. (1998) 'Effectiveness of alliances and partnerships for health promotion', *Health Promotion International*, 13, pp. 99-120.

Hall, P., Brockington, I., Levings, J. and Murphy, C. (1993) 'A comparison of responses to the mentally ill in two communities', *British Journal of Psychiatry*, 162, pp. 99-108.

Homefirst Community Trust (1998) *Rural Health and Social Wellbeing: Making the Connections*, Homefirst Community Trust.

Hope, A., Kelleher, C. C., Holmes, L. and Hennessy, T. (1998) *Health and safety practices among farmers and other workers: A needs assessment*, (under review).

MacDonald, G. and O'Hara, K. (1998) *Ten Elements of Mental Health. Its Promotion and Demotion: Implications for Practice*, Society of Health Education and Health Promotion Specialists, U.K.

Secker, J. (1998) 'Conceptualizations of mental health and mental health promotion', *Health Education Research*, 13, pp. 57-66.

Sogaard, A. and Fonnebo, V. (1995) 'The Norwegian Mental Health Campaign in 1992. Part 2: changes in knowledge and attitudes', Health Education Research, 10 (3), pp. 267-278.

Acknowledgements

The authors of this report gratefully acknowledge the support and assistance of all those who participated in the study. In particular, the Advisory Group of Rural Community Development and Health Project; Mr. Patrick Newe, Director of Adult Services; Dr. Maureen Watson, Head of Mental Health; Mrs. Mary O'Neill, Health Promotion Manager with Homefirst Community Trust, Ms. Felicity Hasson, Research Assistant, University of Ulster at Jordanstown. Colleagues at the Centre for Health Promotion Studies, NUI, Galway, are also thanked, in particular Dr. Ann Hope, Ms. Jane Sixsmith and Professor Cecily Kelleher. The research assistants who collected the data and the community respondents who gave of their time and opinions are also gratefully acknowledged.

2 Mental Health Promotion

Dr. D.R. BILLINGTON

It is a pleasure to be able to speak with you today on the promotion of mental health which is a field central to my technical responsibility in WHO Geneva. This conference will be my first chance to meet some of the leaders of mental health promotion in Europe and I look forward to the next few days to do this.

My presentation today has three objectives:

- first, to comment on what comprises promotion of mental health;
- second, to comment on national infrastructures to promote mental health at national level and
- third, to highlight some priorities for mental health promotion today.

Over the last year I have read with interest the deliberations of several European countries including the United Kingdom to define a framework for action to promote mental health and to discuss the priorities which they see as being of central importance to them. The seriousness and thoroughness of these deliberations are clear to read in the documents that have been produced. While promoting mental health is not a new field of endeavour, the authors have grasped its real importance for our time. Placing the promotion of mental health as one of the two priorities of the Finnish Governments during its tenure in 1999 as chair of the EC is also testimony to the importance.

What Comprises Mental Health Promotion?

There are still differences of opinion among experts about what comes under the umbrella of mental health promotion and whether it includes mental disorder prevention or not. Consensus has not been reached nationally, regionally or globally. More clarity and agreement on what constitutes mental health promotion is needed in order to plan and implement more effective and efficient programmes within countries as well as among those countries, such as those of the European Community, that are attempting to develop international initiatives for mental health promotion involving inter-country governance, legislation and funding.

The experts do seem to agree however, that mental health is an essential and integral component of individual health. This is clearly stated in the WHO definition of health as "a state of complete physical, mental and social well-being and not merely the absence of disease and infirmity". The definition implies that you cannot have health without mental health. It implies that mental health is more than mental disorder.

There is insufficient time in this talk this morning to present fully the promotion/prevention debate, and I am not certain I could do it justice. However, my current view is that mental health promotion comprises the promotion of mental well-being plus the prevention of mental and social problems not classified as mental illnesses. Mental health promotion should also advocate that mental disorder be accorded the same status and empathy as physical disorders, free of stigma and prejudice. But it should not be directly concerned with the prevention of specific mental illnesses. Why?

Mental illness usually refers to recognised medically diagnosed conditions that result in serious disruption of an individuals cognitive, affective and relational abilities, and his or her capacity to live a normal life. Some mental illnesses show a fairly clear separation from normal, such as schizophrenia and Alzheimer's dementia. Others seem to represent the extreme end of a continuum from normal, such as severe depression and obsessive/compulsive disorders. These disorders cannot usually be related to specific experiences of life events. Causation and therefore primary prevention probably lies largely with genetics and biochemistry. As yet we know little that can be applied in practice to prevent these illnesses. Hence mental illness prevention efforts from a behavioural perspective will not be useful.

But there are many less dramatic mental health problems with some disturbance of thought, feeling or behaviour to which the illness model does not apply. These problems are often related to specific negative experiences of physical, personal relationships or life events. They can be perceived as variations or exaggerations of normal experience or normal reactions to life events and circumstances. There is no clear dividing line between "normal" and "abnormal" and the duration of the problem is as important as the severity. A good example is depression and anxiety, sometimes separate, often combined. It is normal to be anxious before an important challenge in life, and normal to be depressed after an important loss or failure. It is also normal to cope with these reactions usually with the help of family and friends and to recover equanimity after a short time. The promotion of mental health includes promoting ways and means for people to cope with these normal problems and in doing so avoid labelling which often accompanies medical care and exacerbates the problem driving it to become a more serious condition. If the reaction is unusually severe or lasts a long time, or counter productive coping methods such as overuse of drugs or alcohol then there is a need for additional help and we have moved from prevention to care.

It is clear then that mental health is not simply the absence of mental disorder but a state of well being in which the individual realises his or her own abilities, can cope with the normal stresses of life, can work productively and fruitfully, and is able to contribute to his or her community. It is also clear that providing for the needs of people with definable mental disorders and promoting mental health in the population are overlapping but very different issues which require to be addressed in different ways.

The Organisation of Mental Health Promotion

I believe that there is consensus for the need for special governmental focus on promoting mental health. Central planning and advocacy is important. Practical and effective collaborative links of the central unit to the implementers of mental health promotion activities, within the Health Department and other government services are essential (such services include education, social work, housing, environment, transport, industry and trade unions, police and justice; and to non governmental or community based organisations, health support groups, the church, charities, societies, clubs and other groups) are also essential.

The special government focal unit for promoting mental health needs to have the freedom to criticise government about existing and proposed policies and practices which conflict with the public mental health. It must have the mandate to propose to government specific activities which will promote mental health. In order to carry out these tasks the focal unit must also have the ways and means to assess and investigate aspects of public mental health.

(In the past the Health Education Authority of England, Wales and Northern Ireland was constantly at odds with government on issues of tobacco control and the Authority was constitutionally changed as a result of this.)

A special authority or counsel located in the health service is usually the focus. Because of the commonality between the aims and tools of general health promotion and mental health promotion some countries opt for the mental health promotion focus to be part of the health education authority. This designation makes sense when one considers the interdependence of physical, social, and mental health, and where one does not want the promotion of mental health to be tainted by psychiatry (see Orley & Birrell Weisen, in press). In some countries there are established health promotion units operating at provincial district level which can incorporate the promotion of mental health into their responsibilities and other services at provincial/district level. If the mental health service gives highest priority for its limited funds to care and allocates little to mental health promotion, which is not an unusual scenario, then it might be advantageous for mental health promotion to join the health promotion authority.

Of course this latter argument presupposes that the health education authority will be committed to the promotion of mental health, and will indeed allocate a fair share of its limited funds and staff to the endeavour. The relative prestige of the health promotion authority and the mental health service is another consideration in their affiliation. Will health promotion taint mental health? That is to say, that if health promotion is not perceived as strong and effective then mental health promotion might be tarred with the same brush.

There are several advantages of having mental health promotion within the mental health service too. There is a growing cadre of mental health professional who have become interested and committed to promoting mental health. This seems to be especially true in Europe where the upsurge of interest in mental health promotion is being lead in part by mental health professionals. There are differences among these professionals as to what constitutes promotion of mental health, as there are among health promotion people. But enthusiasm and agreement among peers can develop with responsibility.

It is not unusual to have prevention and promotion expertise within different departments of a health service where a concentrated effort is needed in a specific priority area. Examples include health education expertise within nutrition services or maternal and child health services or environmental health services. These special focused units help ensure special technical input into promotion and ensure that the service does not abrogate its natural prevention and promotion roles, on the pretence that they are not responsible any more, that promotion and disease prevention is someone else's job. But by not putting mental health promotion into the mental health services it can be interpreted to mean that a mental health service is just for mental health care thus reinforcing the public perception that mental health is indeed mental illness.

Or, could the promotion of mental health be best achieved through the combination of an independent authority external to government involved in reviewing and advocating national mental health policy, but with strong collaborative counterparts in the mental health service at central and provincial levels which have practical links to the other important sectors of government and the community, thus making mental health the responsibility of many.

The foregoing has presented some of the arguments and options to be considered in assessing or reorganising the infrastructure for mental health promotion. There is no best way because all countries differ.

Priorities in Mental Health Promotion

Now I would like to return to the document produced by STAKES summarising the January 1998 Consultative Meeting on Promotion of Mental Health on the European Agenda which was held in Finland. The following 7 strategies or tracks were agreed:

- enhancement of the value and visibility of mental health;
- mental health promotion for children and adolescents;
- mental health promotion, working life and employment;
- mental health promotion and the ageing population;
- social integration of severely marginalised groups (including alcohol and drug misusers);
- development of mental heath indicators;
- telematics and health promotion.

I understand that working groups are now elaborating these tracks in preparation for the high level meeting proposed for the European Community for Autumn 1999. These paths are basic but broad. But if there is a clear focus on selected priorities, then there will be a better chance of mounting and achieving an effective programme. There lurks the danger of trying to do too much in mental health promotion and to be all things to all people which could dilute impact.

What are Some Practical Priorities?

To enhance the value and visibility of mental health may best be attempted through two principal activities. Underlying many mental health problems is poverty and chronic social adversity. There is, therefore, a need for each country to have a national mental health policy which is not solely concerned with mental illness issues but recognises the broader issues affecting all aspects of society and addresses them in ways that are practical within that society. Mental health promotion must be clearly articulated and part of mental health policy. The other important priority in this strategy is to make a concerted effort to remove fear from the word mental and stigma from the term mental illness. It will require a long term effort. Colleagues have suggested that in the meantime, until the meaning of the word mental is neutralised, that the promotion of mental health should drop the phrase mental health and use promotion with a reference to the particular activity being promoted e.g. promoting psychosocial development of children or promoting life skills or promoting child friendly schools, or promoting self esteem etc. But still would remain the overall problems of stigma and fear associated with the word mental and the terms mental health and mental illness which needs a concerted public education to overcome.

Mental Health Promotion for Children and Adolescents is Essential

Early childhood psychosocial development essentially means proper parenting, which means teaching young adults how to be good parents, even providing state support where necessary so they can fulfil this function. I estimate that between 10 to 20% of new mothers are unable to nurture their child and provide the basic love, communication and stimulation needed for the sound emotional and cognitive development of their babies. The implication for secondary education, nursing and welfare services are clear. While there are several benefits for the mother and family, for her to be working outside of the home, there are also disadvantages, unless alternative suitable provision is made. The trend toward single parent families has complicated the problem. Of special concern is the inept single parent without support. Special mental health promotion in this domain is essential.

The school remains a crucial social institution for the education of children not only in numeracy and literacy but also in preparation for life. Schools will need to be more purposively involved in a comprehensive educational role fostering healthy social and emotional development of pupils both inside and outside the classroom. This is the truly comprehensive school; not the one which boasts a wide range of academic subjects. School teachers must be taught to recognise the vulnerable and unhappy child particularly those from dysfunctional families, and know how to handle or refer them discreetly for help. Life skills education should be a significant part of the total school curriculum. Some schools and some teachers make the effort. But not enough. As a priority the agenda for promotion of mental health must include addressing the goals of primary and secondary schooling with education leaders and devising ways to make schools child friendly.

Mental Health Promotion, Working Life and Unemployment Concerns

These usually cover a period of 40 to 50 years. Within this period sits the problems of unemployment for young people and loss of work for those who have family and financial commitments. The effects of poverty and the psychological impact of not having a job on those who want, and who are able, but who cannot get work can be devastating. It is important that mental health promotion examines critically national economic and employment policies and the responsibility of industry to the workforce. The merits of monetarist policies are recognised but the down side of unemployment and the reduction in the quality of life for about 10% of the working population needs attention across many European countries.

Mental Health and the Ageing Population

This is becoming more of an issue as the elderly become a larger percent of the population because people live longer. Ageing is often characterised as biological and physical decline begins after about 30 years of age. But there are important skills and abilities for living which improve with age and experience, and some which reach a certain level in early adulthood and remain well into old age. These include both social and cognitive skills and wisdom. The age of retirement is being debated and greater flexibility is being advocated, somewhat pressured by the problem associated with the provision of pensions. However, I believe that many of the solution to mental health problems of the elderly lie with the elderly. United this group of able people will fare well and generally ensure their own mental well-being and hopefully the well-being of their less competent more vulnerable peers.

The social integration of severely marginalised groups including alcohol and drug users must be a priority for mental health promotion not only because of the misery they inflict on themselves but also the misery they bring to their kin and society. Of particular concern are street children, usually the products of dysfunctional families who have been driven onto the streets and who turn to crime to survive and to drugs to make life immediately bearable. Programmes are required to get these children off the streets to give them the mature adult support most of them need, and to provide mental health care for those already psychologically damaged.

The development of mental health promotion indicators is an important priority, for not only do indicators help in assessing mental health promotion programmes but also provide definable goals for mental health promotion. Indicators influence the emphasis given to the promotion of mental health by the health service. Measures of quality of life and mental well-being are particularly pertinent indicators.

At the beginning of a programme of mental health is a needs assessment, often in the form of an analysis of risk factors and the same assessment is made at the end of the intervention. While these analyses are helpful in designing interventions, they do have the tendency to orient mental health promotion too much towards prevention. An alternative approach may be the assessment of resiliency. Resiliency refers to the capacity to withstand, recover and even grow from the consequences of adversity. Studies of the factors which promote resiliency may help in directing and emphasising what needs to be done to better promote mental health besides studies of risk factors which tend to emphasise prevention of problems.

I hope that this speech has been useful as an introductory activity to this conference. I have tried to be topical and bring your attention to the scope of mental health promotion, some considerations in organising it at national level and some priorities which seem to stand out for continued action. Thank you for listening.

3 Representations of 'Schizophrenia' in Television News: A Comparative Analysis

MIKE BIRCH

The aim of this paper is to explore two television news items on different channels and their depictions of mental health; specifically, two polarised accounts about 'schizophrenia'. The work compares and contrasts the different ways in which each 'order of discourse' structures broadcast journalist discourse and presenter/reporter performance. Examining each item, it investigates how each 'order of discourse' draws normatively and creatively upon each text, working to reshape boundaries and relationships about mental health, or reinforce old ones. Focusing upon key components of 'genre', 'dramatic discourse' and 'visualisations'-'auralisations', the intention is to expose tensions between elements that generate meaning about systems of knowledge and belief. By highlighting representational disparities through the variants of 'understanding' about schizophrenia in news, this critical analysis raises interesting points about how news reports this mental health topic. The two news texts examined are a Channel Four News story entitled 'Schizophrenia Research Appeal' (14/6/93) and an ITN story (7/3/97) about the conviction of a man whose advanced and neglected condition of schizophrenia caused his attempt at several homicides.

Channel Four News and ITN News as 'Genre'

Television news genres operate through codes and conventions, organising programme form. News forms employ studio and location modes of address, using a seated presenter followed by a reporter with direct address, interviews, filmed expositions etc. and through these variety of modes, news discourse is ordered.

ITN News at Ten conforms to dominant news codes and conventions; studio and location modes are tightly linked fitting into specified slots. Pacey presenting gives brief exposés, supplying broad frameworks for understanding, then followed by brisk location reports. In this story about attempted homicides, each element from Trevor MacDonald (the presenter) and Eric MacInnes (the reporter) evoke mythical narratives from horror genres via usage of the term 'paranoid schizophrenic'. I contend this term is typical of most news reports about this story type and that, intertextually, its discursive features draw upon ideas about *'the uncontrollable'* and *'the frenzied erratic madman'* linking with 'not an individual specified or identifiable other text, but a more nebulous 'text' corresponding to general opinion' (Fairclough, 1992:121) about schizophrenia; it references knowledge and belief systems about 'dangerousness' and 'violence' toward the general public. Consequently, this whole generic tendency is one towards the mobilisations of moral panic (see Cohen, 1980).

Channel Four News on the other hand develops away from the currently dominant form of news; its institutional convention and location codes raise 'different' expectation about schizophrenia. Channel Four's institutional remit requires it 'cater for tastes, interests and audiences not previously served by ITV, or any other broadcast channel' (ITN, 1990:934); textually embedded in its news form is a tacitly agreed understanding that such an issue will be covered in different way. Also, the location mode of address uses elements of authorial style and intention in what for this story is a mini-documentary lasting fifteen minutes. Hybridising 'news form' with that of 'documentary', it reshapes normative news discourse to creatively reconfigure boundaries about the condition. It uses musical codes and special imaging devices in addition to accessed voice (which I discuss below). Overall, it departs from dominant news form to arrange 'alternative' systems of knowledge and belief, ordering generic components in a way that serves to open out rather than 'close down' meaning about the condition.

The Order of Discourse in 'Dramatic Discourse'

According to Fairclough (1995) the 'order of discourse' in language is constituted at two levels; genre and discourse. A linguistic genre is, 'a use of language associated with and constituting part of some particular social practice' (Fairclough, 1995:56) and this model I extend to 'a use of language *as*

22

dramatic discourse associated with and constituting part of some particular practice'. Discourse, the second of the two constituent components, relates to knowledge and knowledge construction. Again, I extend this to 'language used *as dramatic discourse* from the presenter's point of view' developing Fairclough's (1995) 'order of discourse' model. This model links to ideas about 'personality' which I contend is intensifying in media accounts (see Tolson, 1991 and Fairclough, 1989; 1992; 1995).

Turning first to the studio mode of address, Trevor MacDonald (ITN) and Jon Snow (Channel Four News) integrate normative social practices, indulging 'the personal' not only through expositional but also aesthetic discourses aided by dramatic elements; expressive codes are integral components of personality and presenting style. Storytelling conventions are skilfully applied to camera and visual aesthetic codes, including competencies in paralinguistic ability and facial expression. Both are competent in 'influencing expressiveness' through use of gaze and facial cast, which can change abruptly to alter 'the mood' of a story.

Both MacDonald and Snow implement 'business-like' styles of dramatic discourse; serious and concerned tones constitute each genre's approach to storytelling. However, in different ways particular to each, expressiveness in facial cast plays a major role in the portrayal of schizophrenia. Initially, MacDonald uses an almost expressionless facial cast complemented by a deep cold voice free of any accent except for a style of received pronunciation, with purposeful and finely applied intonations.

1. The man who attacked a group of children with a machete during a school
2. picnic - was sentenced today. Horret Campbell - a paranoid schizophrenic -
3. was sent to a secure mental hospital indefinitely. A judge said Lisa Potts
4. who protected the children, should be given an award. - ITN's Eric
5. MacInnes was in Court.

A warmer treatment is afforded the young woman through an emerging feature in line 3. Here, MacDonald's facial cast changes, expressing a sense of triumph and jubilation for the woman which simultaneously introduces a tension. As Lisa Potts is centralised as the positive focus, the story of schizophrenia is marginalised. This marginalisation is also assisted by phrases like 'the man who attacked' and 'with a machete' expressed with a unemotional and detached emphasis. Signalled is Campbell's indefinite absence from the social world through knowledge of his identity as one now secured in prison, organising a sense of boundaries needed for confinement of the condition. These integral elements augment with the *paranoid schizophrenic* 'nominalization' (see Fairclough, 1992:179) particular to the genre (see above) serving to construct a sensationalised identity for this 'true' story. Consequently, schizophrenia is denied a 'fair' representation, closing down opportunity of knowledge not only about schizophrenia but also at a wider level, about mental health.

In contrast, Jon Snow's style expressively generates a sympathetic mood in his introduction through the use of gaze; his eyes beckon sympathy about the condition. Similar to MacDonald, his approach is purposeful in wanting to get the message across but restrained; it withholds emotional levels but develops a 'personal' sense of the story via his code of concerned seriousness.

1. A major fund raising effort is to be launched later this week to finance a
2. new research offensive into the devastating mental illness - schizophrenia -
3. The Schizophrenia Research Appeal says that current research is woefully
4. under-funded with just one million pounds spent on investigating the causes
5. of the disease annually - this - despite the fact that almost one in every
6. hundred people in this country will contract it - in this special report our
7. Home Affairs Correspondent Robert Parker has been talking to people with
8. the disease and to those who are engaged in the struggle to find its cause and its cure.

The phrase, '*the devastating mental illness - schizophrenia*' (in line 2) is generically coded as concerned, Snow's tone inflecting an emotionally 'moving' aspect about schizophrenia. It promotes a relationship connecting humane subjectivity with a debilitating mental health condition, its discourse articulating a sense here that schizophrenia is a condition with power over the individual, where the identity of the sufferer is seen as subject to it.

Visualisations - Auralisations

In the ITN example the voice-over by Eric MacInnes further presents knowledge about 'violence' and 'uncontrollability' through an elaborate introduction working in conjunction with visualisations.

In the location mode of address, his genre is vociferous and loud in a way similar to a style of telling tales: I mean by this that resonance associated with

24

a child telling of a misdoing of another in his or her voice. The telling appears more important than the action or event.

1. *The end of the school day and for St. Lukes at last - the end of a terrible*
2. *chapter. Horret Campbell must remain indefinitely in a mental hospital. He*
3. *ran amok with this sixteen inch machete indiscriminately slashing at*
4. *toddlers - teachers and parents at a school's teddy bears picnic. Campbell -*
5. *a paranoid schizophrenic - was obsessed with mass murderers Thomas*
6. *Hamilton and Tasmanian gunman Martin Bryant. As he set off to attack the*
7. *children he thought how to emulate his heroes.*

That the individual actually did attempt to take life is not in dispute here, but it is the pure emphasis on the re-dramatisation of action and event that contributes to a 'mood' (see Fairclough, 1995) of '*that awful event....It's so terrible! You'd think they would do something about it don't you?*'. The discourse is silent about any sense of a debilitating medical condition, presupposing Campbell as a person with pre-planning and calculating skills, similar to 'well' people. Schizophrenia is again damned through the news nominalization of 'paranoid schizophrenic' linking it to the generic stereotype mentioned above.

Visualisations in the ITN text centre on the school with some shots at the court house. The children and their teacher receive understandable attention but it is the placement of the visualised weapon at the beginning of the address which locates the story as 'damnatory'. The choice to view the machete and the way it is visualised is instrumental in provoking relationships of fear. A contextualising view sees it displayed in a box before a new visual runs along its entire blade, the voice over of MacInnes matching the imagery with his words '*He ran amok with this sixteen inch machete indiscriminately slashing at toddlers*'. The decision to represent the implement in this way generates intensified meanings of 'dangerousness' raising tensions that the schizophrenic identity is one problematised with aggressive acts toward people. Such ordering of visual discourse closes down any useful opportunity to explain about the condition.

This contrasts with the voice-over by Robert Parker (Channel Four) and the accompanying visualisation. He operates through a documentary evidential mode or testimony style, re-focalising from a sympathetic point of view the visual portrayals. Vocal codes show his style as one mixing '*logical and detached*' with '*considered and concerned*'.

25

1. People with schizophrenia are tormented by frightening and hideous vi-
*   sions*
2. which they can't control. They have a suicide rate many times higher
*   than*
3. the population at large. It's often because they're acutely aware about
*   how*
4. schizophrenia has ruined their lives. It's sometimes because they cannot
5. resist the voices.

Parker's discourse articulates an enabling knowledge about schizophrenia. In conjunction with the genre's 'considered and concerned' code, and wordings give informative data about schizophrenia as a *'process'* adversely affecting the general well being of the person. The social fact of suicides is raised, illuminating an 'alternative' perspective. The programme's discourse of schizophrenia fosters meaning(s), opening out and freeing for interpretation, the sufferer's own social practices, further assisted by visualisations.

In the location mode of address voice-over, visualisation and auralisation creatively facilitate understanding about schizophrenia. Throughout the text a series of black and white dramatised visual metaphors provide informative evidence re-focalised by Parker's contribution. The first is like a 'see', 'hear' and 'speak' problematisation of the condition. Voices are audible but visually hands block a young woman's ears trying resist them; apparent disturbing images are blocked by hands over the eyes and a screaming mouth is witnessed but without any vocalised terror; a sense of the uncontrolled and fragmentary nature of the condition comes across. Accompanied by a cacophony of classical strings-based instruments screeching loudly coupled with drums, a tension is inscribed. The cacophony of music provides a disturbing feel to the images; an aesthetic discourse of powerful uncontrolled forces administer a discomforting feeling about the human subject in distress, subject to the condition's forces. The third and perhaps most illuminating visualisation positions the audience behind a subject, at an oblique angle, allowing viewers a 'look' at the hallucinations of sufferers. With Parker's discourse (see section above) a young woman is seen using the mirror in which to look at herself, except that, intermittently and without warning a selection of video vignettes depicting snakes, scorpions and spiders emerge superimposed in place of the girl's mirrored face. One senses erratic and chaotic thoughts. Through these codes of representation schizophrenic identity is portrayed as that of an unwell human being in a condition quite beyond the control of the person.

Discussion

> .... the content of press and television showed that two-thirds of media references to mental health related to violence and that these negative images tended to receive 'headline treatment while more positive items were largely 'back page' in their profile.... (Philo *et al.*, 1996:112).

In the light of the above analyses, it is clear that the ITN exemplar falls within that two thirds of negative media identified by Philo *et al.* and that the Channel Four News text is located with the minority. The former illuminates the schizophrenic identity as a kind of outlaw culture through its projected systems of beliefs and knowledge; it produces the stereotype of a 'dangerous and fearful *other*' raising parallels with how other social groups have been oppressed in media. Similarities with the homosexual group abound (see Morrison in Hargrave, 1992) but likewise raise implications about the formation of identity if their subjectivity is one whose mentality is, not only misrepresented in the symbolic universe of everyday media representation, but also rarely reported accurately. Questions are raised about what ramifications arise for those whose mentality, if already damaged, are then further subjected to highly publicised impoverished ideas about their identity. Evidently, the Channel Four News text details facts in a way according with studies such as that by Häfner and Bröker (1973) and the report by Boyd (1996), both of which clearly articulate the situation for the schizophrenic as one more likely to be injurious to their own self than to others. With little or no public profile in terms of major campaign groups like that of gay, ethnic and other marginalised groups, it would appear this social group has yet to find its voice in society, their contemporary situation best described as 'a discourse of silence'. How might news policy change in order to better represent these people and the concept of mental health in general?

Conclusion

Each news text's discourse is ordered using a variety of components in ways which imply one or other perspective about the condition of schizophrenia. Clearly, homicides rate highly in news values as 'dramatic' and therefore, 'dramatically' reportable stories, the ITN example being a case in point. Generic implications arise in the term 'paranoid schizophrenic' and visualisations of weapons also raise expectation about mythical meanings. I contend that such linguistic and visual 'dramatisations' incite 'dangerousness and fear'

27

evacuating understanding and wherever possible, such representations should be avoided. Instead, 'personality' could be dramatically employed in conjunction with 'language' depicting mental health in ways which raise awareness. In news media generally, the topic of counselling is one example where nearly all forms operate a strongly sympathetic policy exacted to subjects who are victims (or relatives of victims) in tragedies such as a train crash. In the studio mode of address, the presenter's voice dips and a sympathetic gaze, typically encourages 'understanding' for those caught up in the accident and who will need counselling. In my opinion, this re-presenting process draws in new understanding about mental health, inviting inquiry and therefore interest about associated issues. It elevates the issue of mental health above institutional need of a good story, locating it as an important and sensitive concept worthy of careful representational codes.

I believe the key to problems about representing schizophrenia to be a simple one. By following the information put forward by the Boyd Inquiry (and that data put forward by Häfner and Bröker), accurate knowledge might inform understanding about schizophrenia. If news institutions were to reduce those generic elements that mobilise moral panic instead of illuminating understanding, and employ more often codes like those articulated in the Channel Four example, new understanding about the issue of schizophrenia and about mental health generally might have space to emerge. Of course, this 'if' perhaps begs some rather large questions about the current factors underlying the 'popular' in TV news.

References

Boyd, W. *(1996) Report of the Confidential Inquiry into Homicides and Suicides by Mentally Ill People,* Royal College of Psychiatrists.

Cohen, S. *Folk Devils and Moral Panics* (1980) Martin Robertson, Oxford.

Fairclough, N. *(1989) Language and Power,* Longman.

Fairclough, N. *(1995) Media Discourse,* Edward Arnold.

Fairclough, N. *(1992) Discourse and Social Change,* Polity.

Häfner and Bröker (1973) *Crimes of Violence by Mentally Abnormal Offenders. A psychiatric and epidemiological study in the Federal German Republic* (trans, Marshall, H., 1982).

ITN Fact Book (1990) Michael O'Mara Books Ltd.

Morrison, D. (1992) in A. M. Hargrave, *Sex and Sexuality in Broadcasting,* Broadcasting Standards Council, John Libbey.

Philo, G. (ed.) *(1996) Media and Mental Distress,* Longman.

Tolson, A.(1991) in Scannell, P. (ed.) *Broadcast Talk,* Sage.

4 Promoting Mental Health in Media: in Search of an Effective Methodology

MIKE BIRCH

This working paper is part of a Ph.D. process and constitutes work toward completion of an audience reception study entitled The Representation of Mental Health in Media at the University of Liverpool.

Introduction

Across the last forty years a range of studies has examined mental health and illness, and the media's role in the formulation of public beliefs and attitudes about it. Most, if not all, focus on the understanding of negative issues (questions linked to dangerousness, crime and risk) whilst some, very few, provide more positive data or perspectives. A recent study by Philo et al. (1996) provides useful findings but again, still addresses mainly negative issues about mental health coverage in media. This book, another by Otto Wahl (1995), research by Atkinson (1995), Birch (1997) and Hyler et al. (1991) seeks social change in media representations about mental health, all part of a growing body of evidence signalling a clear and serious need for modification of media policy. The weight of evidence does, if anything, indicate urgent need to actively develop a 'methodology' promoting understanding of mental health at a time when facilitating cultural acceptance and understanding is a key to enabling positive social change. Therefore, this paper reviews previous studies into mental health and media, with the intention of searching for useful strategies to assist methodology development. Its focus selects and examines previous, and recently developed work, advancing perspectives of inquiry

29

which best serve mental health promotion. Consequently, rather than keeping the study trapped within negatively-inclined procedures, consideration in the search is afforded to interpretative methodologies, one being awarded special attention.

Reviewing Critically, Secker and Platt's 'Critical Research Review'

In *Media and Mental Distress* (Philo, 1996) Secker and Platt critically review a range of research studies. In their chapter, '*Why Media Images Matter*', two sections explore research, the first examining how British mass media portray mental illness investigating media image content whilst the second reviews previous research into the impact of the media images on public attitudes and beliefs. As Secker and Platt's work shows, little is known about the part media plays in shaping public beliefs as there is a scarcity of research assessing the impact of media images, either positive or negative on beliefs and attitudes. Their purpose was to supply some contextualising data in order to determine the significance of the research, their aim, to 'provide a systematic analysis of the way in which British mass media portray mental health issues' and, 'to develop research methods which would allow us to explore the complex processes involved in the interpretation of media messages', Philo et al. (1996:17). From *Media and Mental Distress*, I select several methodologies for review; one by Belson (1967), another by Wober (1989), as these suggest media coverage can be beneficial in impact, and two by Philo (1996). Because of space restrictions, Philo's work is the main focus in this examination, which avoids where possible discussion about findings.

Belson and Wober: Method Reflections

Belson (1967), examined the impact of one television documentary series (in 1956), *The Hurt Mind*, on viewers' ideas and attitudes about mental health issues; six programmes covered a range of perspectives connected with mental illness, particularly perceptible causes and different methods of attending to them. Wober (1989) examined the effects of a Channel Four Mental Health 'campaign' between 1st October to 21st November in 1986; twelve programmes were broadcast including three entitled, *Living With Schizophrenia*. The main study intention was to 'discover something about the attitudes of viewers towards people with mental health problems or disturbance, and to see what kinds of attitudes relate with viewing more or less of the set of programmes' (1989:3).

Each method took account of demographic variables of age, gender and class but utilised different approaches to producing data. In Belson's method, after respondents had viewed the second, third, fourth and/or fifth programme, special recruiting procedures[1] drew together large groups (45 people) in one large room for questioning by a single interviewer. Viewers and non-viewers of the series were invited without foreknowledge of study content and asked to write down answers to questions without discussion. Questions aided three purposes: First, 'whether or not it was necessary to spend program time in correcting images and in softening attitudes' Belson (1967:76); second, that 'they should identify the kinds of information that most lacked (with respect to type, causes and treatment of mental illness) so that the effort to inform them might be most efficiently focused' (ibid:76); and finally that 'they should help the producer to avoid showing things especially upsetting to the viewer' (ibid:76). Wober's methodology involved respondents from a Broadcasters' Audience Research Board panel of viewers, based on a nationally representative sample. Keeping a diary, respondents recorded answers to a list of questions in a booklet along with other questions about television. Statements supplemented by questions worded in a positive and negative sense to balance for 'leading' opinion were presented. The first statement was about 'attitudes towards mental ill health: the mentally ill'; the second, 'attitudes towards mental ill health: social closeness'; the third about, 'attitudes towards mental ill health programmes: identification and effects'. Measurements were applied, additional calibrations linking resulting variables, informed further critical findings.

Both Wober and Belson provide useful method lessons in 'social context' and 'genre'. Each procedure avoids 'genre recognition', denying the critical division between fictional and non fictional television programmes and the knowledge properties that stem from each; a research point made by John Corner (1991) in an essay examining the problematics of 'public knowledge' in new audience studies. Here, he critiques previous research, raising questions about:

> *what* meanings audiences make of what they see, hear and read, *why* these meanings rather than others are produced by specific audiences from the range of interpretative possibilities, and *how* these activities of meaning-making, located as they usually are in the setting of everyday domestic life, might relate to ideas about power of the media and about the constitution of public knowledge, sentiment and values.
>
> Corner (1991:267)

Future strategies could focus critically upon the kinds of knowledge or pleasure resident in generic forms about mental health facilitating more in-depth and specific information; particularly from a one genre study, such as Belson's, no less value being accorded a multiple genre study like Wober's. Also, method might adopt more critical approaches to 'situate' acts of viewing in their 'social context', another area of analysis which Corner argues needs tightening-up at its 'edges'. Toward methodological development, he divides this element into two contextual realms, *social relations*[2] of viewing and *space/time settings.*[3] In developing social relations, he identifies 'variations in disposition and 'cultural competence' (including familiarity with particular linguistic and aesthetic conventions) which occur *within* as well as between the conventional sociological categorizations' (1991:278). Types or experience of occupation groups like carers, survivors of 'Care in the Community', broadcast journalists, builders, etc.,would be worth exploration. Also useful are, 'theme-specific categories', where viewer accounts about 'health' meanings might inform different and varying patterns from those about 'illness'; these would, I think, yield useful social findings about different interpretative reactions. Additionally, 'situated' viewing in *space* and *time* contexts could delineate further, motives and rituals around watching mental health texts and viewer relationships; as in why people do and don't attend to mental health specific generic forms and *how* they do.

Philo's Study: Method, Reflection, Development

Philo's methods were developed after examination of the above and other studies. Purposefully, both service and non service-users of mental health care services were included in two separate methods. A nation-wide service-user interview study took place at drop-in centres, whilst six small focus groups constituted the non service-user group study; they were broadly representative of earning levels, job and housing class or type for the area of the west of Scotland and randomly chosen.

Users were sensitively approached in small groups; discussion opened out issues about media images and their stigmatising nature. Highly structured and open-ended questions inquired about *change* in user belief and attitudes *before* and *after* diagnosis of unwell mental health; their focus 'public attitudes to mental illness and the sources of information which underpinned people's beliefs and emotional responses' (1996:106). Inquiry sought reaction to their condition as well as reflection about new personal belief. Confidentiality, the most important qualifier in undertaking this study was maintained in terms of name, date and place of interview. The non-user study main aim inquired of people's expectations about what they would see in media as well as their understanding and memory of particular styles of output; it examined the interpretative processes by which beliefs and attitudes develop. Through a process of 'writing the news' for two printed news media, one positive 'achievement' story (a former patient achieving status as one of the top five learners in Scotland) and one associated with dangerousness (later disclaimed by media), non-users were asked to write and develop their own story from a given newspaper headline. Another process of 'writing the dialogue' for a fictional programme Coronation Street (a soap opera) drew out member's own ideas, creatively calling upon a range of responses relative to dialogue, character and plot structure. Given only photographs, members had to reproduce dialogue around a negativised mentally ill character called Carmel. Divided into three specific phases, each group was first split into smaller units of two or three people, and given exercise work in writing a news report or the dialogue for the fictional programme (i.e. a soap opera). Exercises were identified as having an important function, facilitating a collective activity in which people could begin to express their own ideas in a relatively informal way; an attempt to produce 'natural' responses in people; secondly, a series of answers to questions focused on belief about mental illness and the sources of such beliefs; and third, individuals were later interviewed in-depth about their own answers. Two questions were constructed for these exercises but there were also other questions designed as indicators of sources of beliefs about mental illness. One question looked at what media content might be with three others inquiring as to how content might relate to the development of belief.

Both methods are crucial to understanding user and non-user interpretative processes and *what* 'meanings' they read in media messages about mental health/illness and *why*. Central to Philo's findings, particularly about service-users, are *social identity* and *relationships* of difference (see Philo, 1996:108-111), around which *more* in-depth clarification could have facilitated clearer recognition of 'life-worlds'. 'Meaning making' (and meaning per se in the areas covered above), require clarity which Corner, again, identifies as a problematic area in reception analysis for both interpretation and textual signification. Offering '*levels*' as a narrowing device for the phenomena under study, the first level resembles denotation, 'a word, image or sequence's primary signification' (1991:271) whilst the second, connotation is 'a word, image or sequences' secondary, implicatory or associative signification' (ibid:271). The third level is one attaching:

33

a generalized significance to what they have seen or heard, evaluating it (perhaps in relation to its perceived presuppositions and entailments if it has propositional force) and locating it within a negotiated place in their knowledge or memory, where it may continue to do modifying work on other constituents of their consciousness (and, indeed, of their consciousness).
Corner (1991:272)

Application of this framework as a critical instrument, improves 'meaning making' definition, constricting inference particularly where connotative values propagate a multiplicity of meanings.

The methods designed by Philo *et al.* are both creative and useful, however, on reflection, outcomes suggest reinforcement of previous findings and concerns; fears that the social impact of media representations on service-users *are* a worry, worthy of further serious consideration (Vousden, 1989; Birch, 1991; Hyler et al, 1991; Atkinson, 1994). It follows that the need for an 'effective methodology' promoting mental health becomes all the more imperative and a search *must* enable *social change* not only for service-users but also society more broadly. Therefore, I propose a strategy which combines the work of Paulo Freire (1970) and drama, developing a method of 'media community drama': Using critically the processes of drama, service-users investigate mental health meanings in media employing drama as a tool with which to develop social change in the community; this, achieved via a process of *conscientisation*, which I now explain.

Central to Freire's *conscientisation* method is the process whereby *change* occurs through participant investigation; users perform the inquiry themselves rather than it being done by the expert. A preliminary meeting with users, proposes sensitively the area for examination and discussion, raising awareness of the key method elements of 'language' *and* 'the dramatic' in language, narrative, character, image and/or sound organising concepts of social identity and relations. Across three phases of reception, interpretation and production small groups process media texts with a view to development. As objects of problematic media representations at the reception stage users explore generated themes, searching stories implying myths and/or notions of dangerousness. Here, each media text is what Freire (1970) terms an 'untested feasibility' in which user-perception and knowledge, although raised by searching for problematic elements is in a 'limit situation'; this situation requiring a testing of the text by users to facilitate a 'limit act', a liberation from its oppressive shackles. Interpreting textual details elements are *processed* and *transformed*, user-consciousness *raised* stimulating details about their 'reality and self', this testing, changing linguistic and dramatic elements about identity and relations. At the production stage, changed elements are rehearsed for production before camera or microphone, or in writings and photographs before a final production process organises new developed texts which are in Freire's terms a 'potential consciousness'. Users 'act out' interpretations producing new characterisations and dialogue in news presenter communications, documentaries and also, soaps; language and tone are developed suggesting new ways and terms for communicating about mental health. In this way, developing Philo's *writing the news* method in printed, and on-line media facilitates text transformation of the dramatic and the sensationalised (see Day and Page, 1986). Another development of the *Coronation Street* text (see above) focuses upon the character of Carmel which received unfavourable portrayal. Here, re-writing the story-line, re-acting the characterisation and a critical scene could produce new and more informed mental health meaning from the user-perspective. Operating a separate coding system for language and dramatic elements, evaluation of findings are subject to reduction by sorting, categorisation and interrelation of variables according to emerging schemas (see Lindlof, 1995). Through a quantitative and qualitative procedure, linguistic and dramatic elements are identified providing new terms and new ways in which to communicate terms. A follow-up process engaging reflexivity in another user-group, assesses findings, enhancing validity and reliability to yield a trustworthy set of results. Finally, presenting non-users with a sequence of the original and then user-developed texts could focus their responses, locating initial and then developed beliefs and attitudes. This might usefully expose the processes of 'changing' beliefs and attitudes for a more critical understanding.

Concluding Recommendations

In view of this somewhat fragmented analyses, I will conclude by drawing together searched strategies in an 'experimental' block of study recommending a potentially effective method. In a reception study of both service and non service-users groups, a range of texts are presented for interpretation. Operating a genre sensitive framework across 'demographic' and 'special interest' organised groups facilitates an accurate and informed typology; this process also taking account of 'situated' viewing to inform more focused diverse and specific data about mental health knowledge. Applying a strict framework of '*levels*' across methods would constrict sloppy inference in this and the following study stage. Next, users, through a form of 'media community drama' examines media texts organising counter images of mental health through the processes of *conscientisation* by their receiving, interpreting and producing 'developmental' pieces; these for assessment by both user and non-user groups, the latter give focused reliability and validity in findings, the former facilitating data about attitudes and beliefs in respect of these texts prior to, and post, user-interventions. Through this methodology a key mode communication is utilised, the critical power of drama (in a media dramatised world) engaging with problematic mental health meanings to supply a way forward promoting new understanding. By engaging public belief not only about the plight of people who suffer mental health problems but also, in a future project, illuminating a wider potential 'for a mentally healthier way of life'. By taking these methods forward, and utilising the critical power of drama, promotion of mental health in media could help comprehension about ill-health, developing public knowledge and encouraging changed beliefs and attitudes.

References

Atkinson, J. M. and Coia, D. A. (1995) *Families coping with Schizophrenia: a model of group work for family support* in Willey, J. (ed.) Families Coping With Schizophrenia, Wiley, Chichester.

Belson, W. (1967) *The Impact of Television: Methods and Findings in Program Research* Crosby and Lockwood and Son Ltd, London.

Birch, J. (1991) *Towards the Restoration of Traditional Values in the Psychiatry of Schizophrenia* Context, 8:21-26.

Birch, M. (1997) *Representations of 'Schizophrenia' in Television News: A Comparative Analysis* unpublished paper from the Seventh Annual European Conference On The Promotion Of Mental Health, Maastricht, 1997.

Corner, J. (1991) *Meaning, Genre and Context: The Problematics of 'Public Knowledge' in the New Audience Studies* in Curran J. and Gurevitch, M. (eds.) Mass media and Society, London, Edward Arnold.

Day, D. and Page, S. (1986) *Portrayal Of Mental Illness in Canadian Newspapers* in the Canadian Journal Of Psychiatry, 31 (December): 813-17.

Freire, P. (1970) *Pedagogy Of The Oppressed* New York, Seabury Press.

Hyler, S. *et al.* (1991) *Homicidal Maniacs and Narcissistic Parasites: Stigmatisation Of Mentally Ill persons in the Movies* Hospital and Community Psychiatry, 42 (10).

Lindlof, Thomas R. (1995) *Qualitative Communication Research Methods* Sage.

Mies, M. in Hammersely, M. (ed.) (1993) *Social Research: Philosophy, Politics and Practice* Sage.

Philo, G. (ed.) (1996) *Media and Mental Distress* Longman.

Secker J. and Platt, S. in Philo, G. (ed.) (1996) *Media and Mental Distress* Longman.

Vousden, M. (1989) *Loony Lefties and Mad Mullahs* Nursing Times, 85 (28):16-17.

Wahl, Otto F. *Media Madness, Public Images Of Mental Illness* Rutgers University Press, 1995.

Wober, J. (1989) *Healthy Minds On Healthy Airwaves: Effects Of Channel 4's 1986 Mental Health Programme Campaign* Independent Broadcasting Authority Research Department, London.

Notes

1 Belson's recruiting procedures are lengthy and detailed. For a more specific account, see *The Impact Of Television* (1967:13-26 and 76-77).

2 For Corner, researchers must ask 'what are the social relations of viewing?' Research design must be developed beyond demographic variables in order to understand the 'complex structures and processes which might bear on the *sociality* of interpretative action' (1991:278).

3 An analysis of the space and time context factors of 'situated viewing', looks at the daily routines and rituals of viewing in order to extract better understanding about the constituent moods, motives and 'rituals' of viewing' (1991:280).

5 Same Sex Attraction in Young People: Health, Happiness and Homophobia

ADRIAN BOOTH

Space boy, you're sleepy now
your silhouette is so stationary
you're released but your custody calls
and I want to be set free
don't you want to be free
do you like girls or boys
it's confusing these days
but moondust will cover you
cover you
this chaos is killing me

(Hallo Spaceboy, Bowie/ Eno, Produced by the Pet Shop Boys, 1995)

Introduction

The journey undertaken by young people who are experiencing same sex attraction is one of complexity, uncertainty and confusion. Young people who are struggling with making sense of their lives face isolation, stigma and rejection from society. Young gay, lesbian, bi-sexual youth are at increased risk of poor social and emotional wellbeing and increasingly research indicates that same sex attraction is a major factor in youth suicide although this interelationship remains controversal (La Barbèra, 1994; Shaffer et al 1995).

This paper will look at the issues and risks that face young gay, lesbian and bisexual youth (hereafter referred to by the letters G LB) and will review

39

some of the available research that has been undertaken. Australian initiatives regarding same sex attraction and suicidal risk prevention programs will be highlighted and a framework for action will be proposed.

In preparing this paper a review of journal and internet site literature has been undertaken which has primarily focussed on GLB youth. However it is acknowledged that young people who are experiencing transgendered issues may also be considered an at risk group as it has been argued that their problems are similar to those experienced by youth who have a minority sexual orientation (Gibson, 1989).

Issues and Risk Factors for Young People Experiencing Same Sex Attraction

A recent forum in Canberrra, Australia revealed that 10 young people kill themselves each week and 60,000 young people attempt suicide each year. In a study which was undertaken with 3000 young people who visited General Practitioners, 1 in 17 had made a serious attempt on their life (Here For Life, Canberra, 1998). It has been argued that Australia has one of the highest suicide rates in the world of which 80% are male and the 16-25year age group are the most vulnerable (Brown, 1996).

As a response to these figures a National Youth Suicide Strategy was initiated which aims to reduce the incidence of youth suicide in Australia (National Youth Suicide Prevention Strategy, 1997). A young person's journey into adulthood can be complex, chaotic and consist of personal and emotional struggles in defining their sense of who they are and how they can achieve an independent place within society (Erickson,1950).

A number of factors influence a young person's social and emotional wellbeing. These include the importance of the family and home environment for protecting adolescents from harm. In addition, young people's health can be influenced by risk taking behaviours which can involve drinking and driving, violence, substance use and unsafe sex. (Add health, 1995).

Depression has been the most frequently reported mental health problem in adolescents and is the single largest risk factor for suicidal behaviour (Shaffer et al, 1996).

Recent reports demonstrate that between 15-40% of young people report depressive symptoms with the highest rates involving the 15-24 year age group (NHMRC, 1997).

The above work has predominately taken place across the general youth population and has not, as a result, focussed on the GLB youth population.

GLB youth are a subgroup of this wider youth population group and according to a review of the current literature would appear initially to share similar characteristics with heterosexual young people. However research on youth suicidality has commonly 'ignored' the relationship of sexual orientation issues and suicidal behaviour in young people. Such a relationship has been discounted due to erroneous research methodology (LaBarbara, 1994; Shaffer et al, 1995; Muehrer, 1995) and problems associated with the homophobia of professionals within the suicidology area (Tremblay,1996).

There is increasing evidence that sexual orientation issues in young people play a predominant role in suicidal behaviour. Issues such as discrimination, coming out, establishing a gay identity, racial and ethnic factors and limited support structures all affect young GLB youth (Millard, 1995). Other studies have found that young GLB people have higher rates of other psychosocial problems including alcoholism, illicit drug use, victimisation and homelessness (Falkner and Cranston, 1998; Remafedi et al, 1991).

Other common issues for young GLB youth have been found to include low self esteem, social isolation, depression, negative family interactions, negative social attitudes, the school and peer group and safe sex issues (Proctor and Groze, 1994; Brown, 1996; Remafedi, 1987a).

Unlike their heterosexual peers it has been argued that GLB youth experience tremendous pressure in denying their same sex preferences and subsequently deny any thoughts, beliefs or actions which may be associated with same sexual attraction issues (Rotheram-Borus, Fernandez, 1995). Gibson (1989) also suggests that young GLB youths face a 'double jeopardy' of surviving the trials of adolescence and also developing a gay identity within a hostile and prejudiced environment. Gibson highlights that gay youth face problems in accepting themselves due to the internalisation of a negative self image and lack of accurate information regarding homosexuality during adolescence. Uribe and Harbech (1992) also assert that a young person experiencing same sex attraction, journeys through adolescence facing negative gay stereotypes and a lack of information on what same sex attraction means. In addition they argue that homophobic attitudes toward young GLB youth have been seen as being similar in content to racist and sexist attitudes.

As the above research shows young GLB people face predjudice, discrimination and possible violence within a society that is largely heterocentric. Therefore the traditional moral values of a society can be a major barrier for GLB youth as highlighted in the following quote.

> Children who should be taught to respect traditional moral values are being taught they have the unalienable right to be gay (Thatcher, 1987 Tory Party Conference).

This moralistic viewpoint has not assisted in reducing the difficulties experienced by GLB youths in England.

Recognition of GLB rights is a continuing issue which challenges notions of what is considered right and just by a dominant heterosexist society. It was not until 1973 that homosexuality was not classified as a mental disorder.

Homosexuality has been a crime punishable by law and attempts to change the law in one of Australia's States, Tasmania, will mean that it is not illegal to be in a homosexual relationship. In England the age of consent for young GLB people to be reduced to 16 years of age has recently been debated within parliament.

Even though there seems to have been some shifts in community attitude towards homosexuality, stigma, hatred and prejudice still remain.

Crucial to a person's emotional and social wellbeing is the perception of belonging or feeling connected to one's environment. In an Australian study, issues surrounding social connectedness and emotional wellbeing have been found to be important for young people (Glover et al, 1998). Students who reported poor social connectedness (having no –one to talk to or no one to trust) are between 2-3 times more likely to experience depressive symptoms when compared to peers who have more positive relationships. Even though this study involved students drawn from a general population base it can be argued that the importance of belonging or connecting with a social group or community is extremely important for young GLB youth.

The above issues suggest that young GLB youth face specific issues which are different from those experienced by heterosexual young people. This factor has tended to be ignored by suicidologists (Tremblay, 1996). There has been increasing research, particularly within the United States, which suggests that same sex attraction should be considered a major risk factor in youth suicide. However this research remains controversial as it has been argued that homosexual activists have manipulated this relationship to further their own political agenda (La Barbara,1994).

In an Australian study, which involved thirty gay young men in Western Australia, Brown (1996) found that over half of the sample had attempted suicide. In addition most had experienced depression, confusion and anxiety. The actual process of discovering their sexuality and dealing with the community's values impacted on their relationships, ability to communicate and self esteem. Hammelman in 1993 suggested that GLB youth are at increased risk of suicide if they:

- discover their same sex preference early in adolescence;
- experience violence due to their gay or lesbian identity;

- use drugs or alcohol to cope with problems regarding their sexual orientation;
- are rejected by family members as a result of being gay or lesbian.

The process of 'coming out' for young GLB people has been an integral part of the discussions within past and current research.

Given the stigma and taboos contained within our society it remains difficult for young people to talk openly to others, friends, family or school counsellors through fear of being rejected or ridiculed. Thus a form of self imposed isolation develops where internal battles take place around what sexuality you 'should' be as opposed to what sexuality you 'feel' you are. This internal struggle comes at a time where young people are trying to make sense of their identity.

There have been attempts to develop stages of coming out (Kus, 1980; Rotheram-Borus and Fernandez, 1995) ie, recognizing oneself as GLB, disclosing to others and becoming more comfortable with accepting one's sexual orientation are all integral steps that young GLB people can experience in coming to terms with their same sex attraction.

Work undertaken by Rotheram- Borus and Fernandez has been criticised by Olsen and King (1995) who argue that the coming out process may infact be influenced by a whole range of influences which include family, personal or cultural experiences and therefore not soley influenced by being attracted to same sex peers.

There has been much debate regarding the role that same sex attraction plays in suicidal behaviour in young people. Much of this debate centres around unsound methodology including the recognised absence of comparison groups (Faulkner and Cranston, 1998); lack of carefully designed studies (Moscicki, 1995) or lack of any 'real' evidence (Muehrer, 1995; Shaffer et al, 1995; LaBarbara, 1994). Such debate is beyond the scope of this paper however it is appearing increasingly likely that same sex attraction is a major factor in GLB youth suicide and GLB young people are at increased risk of attempting suicide when compared to heterosexual young people. Table 1 attempts to summarise some of the studies undertaken on GLB youth suicide.

These studies highlight the increasing importance of the role that same sex attraction in young people plays in relationship to suicidal behaviour. The controversial nature of such a relationship by some authors has been highlighted however it appears that with the range of studies undertaken and with an improved emphasis on research methodology including design, meas-

Table 1 Review of Studies Focussing on GLB Youth Suicide

Author	Subjects	Findings
Bagley & Tremblay (1997) (USA)	750 males (age 18-27)	homosexual men 13.9 times more at risk of serious suicide (process of coming out highlighted as possible link)
Bell & Weinberg (1978) (USA)	575 homosexual men; 284 heterosexual (matched)	homosexual men 13.6 times more likely to have attempted suicide prior to 21men
Brown (1996) (Australia)	30 out of 100 17-29 young men identified as Gay or Bisexual	23 out of 30 contemplated suicide 17 out of 30 attempted suicide
Faulkner & Cranston (1998) (USA)	using 93 sample of 3054 grade 9-12 students in Massachusetts	homosexuality active adolescents 4.2 times more likely to have attempted suicide compared to heterosexual adolescents
Garofalo et al (1998) (USA)	using random sample of 4159 grade 9-12 students using Masch's youth risk survey, 1995	GLB youth 3.6 times more likely to attempt suicide than non GLB youth
Kruks (1991) (USA)	using data from unpubl'd study- 53 gay identified street youths	53% had attempted suicide at least once
Remafedi et al (1998) (USA)	used 1987 sample of 36,254 Minno'ta grade 7-12 students	GLB students 7 times more at risk of attempting suicide compared to heterosexual youths
Youth risk behaviour survey, Seattle (1996) (USA)	8400 grade 9-12 students	GLB students were 3 times as likely to have attempted suicide 12 months prior to the survey
Youth risk behaviour survey, Masch's (1995) (USA)	3054 grade 9-12 students	GLB students 4 times more likely to have attempted suicide in past year
Youth risk behaviour survey, Vermont (1995) (USA)	grade 8-12 students	GLB students 2.5 times more likely to have attempted suicide in past year

* note studies of Garofalo et al (1998) and Faulkner and Cranston (1998) found GLB young people more likely to engage in drug use, alcohol use, miss school and experienced sexual assault as compared to non GLB young people.

44

urement and sampling methods, the rejection of the role of same sex attraction in preventing youth suicide is becoming less salient.

Future Directions

Australian Initiatives and a Framework for Action

There are a number of initiatives that are being undertaken in Australia at present. All of these interventions are based on the goal to reduce suicidal behaviour in young people who are sexually attracted to their same sex. The Western Australian Here for Life, Youth Sexuality project (1996) aims to:

- target young people whose suicidal behaviour is linked to their same sex attraction;
- design key prevention strategies which modify suicidal behaviour and attitudes whilst focussing on sexuality issues;
- developing these target and prevention strategies into a best practice model and forming effective partnerships with mainstream services in the community.

Across Australia a project entitled 'What turns you on?' has surveyed youth via the internet and youth appropriate magazines. This survey included a range of questions which looked at, for example, knowledge, sexual behaviour and basis of attraction. Results of the survey will be available in November (Walsh and Hillier, 1998). In South Australia a project entitled 'Don't take your life-Celebrate it' will be commencing shortly. This project will aim to reduce the incidence of suicidal behaviour among young people with same sex attractions by:

- improve the knowledge and referral practices of mainstream services;
- increasing the knowledge and skills of parents;
- raising the awareness of support services available to young GLB youth in SA.

A useful framework for action that has been highlighted (Brown,1996) is the Ottawa Charter (1986). The five action areas of the Charter provide a useful health promotion framework for intervention and a way of planning

45

effective and appropriate programs taking into account the complex factors that influence health.

Building Healthy Public Policy

The Public Health Sector needs to ensure that the issue of same sex attraction in young people and its relationship to suicidal behaviour is integrated with all aspects of youth policy particularily those which address suicide prevention strategies. In addition, it is important that all mental health promotional and policy material be openly inclusive of GLB issues and co-ordinated across the health sector (Report of South Australian Working Party,1997).

Strengthening Community Action

Taking collective action around HIV/AIDS is a good example of how the GLB community(ies) has tackled this issue and responded by reducing the incidence of HIV.It has been suggested that much of the emphasis on young GLB people has stemmed from the HIV related programs which can however restrict the focus away from broader issues (Brown, 1996). These issues may involve violence, homophobia and addressing the lack of role models for GLB youth. Young GLB people's involvement in addressing these areas reaffirms their role as active citizens of society and can help to reduce their sense of isolation.

Developing Personal Skills

Developing the skills of GLB young people regarding issues of acceptance, promoting a strong sense of identity and providing information regarding support agencies is vital in reducing at risk and suicidal behaviours. Utilising peer support has been argued to be the cornerstone of successful behaviour change as it promotes healthy behaviour while affirming a young persons identity (Goggin and Sotiropoulos, 1994). We also need to ensure that health and human services workers who work with suicidal youth are aware of the issues of same sex attraction (Kourany, 1987).

Creating Supportive Environments

Environments that engender safety, respect and recognition of difference will provide environments of support to young GLB people. The importance of connectedness with one's surroundings has been shown to be vital (Glover et al, 1998). The availability of positive role models,for example, Ian Roberts a recently identified gay man who is a Australian rugby league player and Rob Halford ex lead singer of Heavy metal band Judas Priest help to 'normalise' gay behaviours and provide a much needed role model for young GLB people. Recommendations from the Safe Schools Anti Violence Documentation Project (1996) reinforces the importance of safe, supportive school environments through education and preventing homophobia.

Re-orientating Health Services Toward Prevention

Ensuring that issues relating to the health and wellbeing of young GLB people are incorporated into the human services sector is an important strategy to undertake. Dispelling myths and stereotypes around homosexuality and recognising and challenging homophobia within the workplace will result in health promoting services which young GLB people can access. It has been argued that educational efforts, prevention programs and health services must be designed to address the unique needs of GLB youth (Garofalo et al, 1998).

This paper has attempted to capture the current issues and research surrounding the emerging evidence of the role that same sex attraction has in regard to youth suicide. Whilst the majority of research promotes the view of young GLB people being at increased risk of suicide this relationship requires further scrutiny through sound methodological enquiry particularily within an Australian context where research on same sex attraction and it's relationship to suicidal behaviour is scarce.

This paper has not debated the issue of population based estimates of homosexuality. Neither has it looked at the differences between gay and bisexual males and lesbian and bi-sexual females. These topics are beyond the scope of this paper however they are important components of building an overall picture of same sex attraction in young people and the relationship to suicidal behaviour.

References

Add Health (1997) 'National Longitudinal study of Adolescent Health Youth Studies Australia', pp. 37-50, December.

Bagley, C., Trembley P. (1997) 'Suicidal behaviours in homosexual and bisexual males', *Crises*, 18 (1), pp. 24-34.

Bell A. P., Weinberg M. S. (1978) *Homosexualities: A study of diversity among Men and Women*, Simon and Schuster, New York.

Brown, G. (1996) 'Sexuality issues and risk taking behaviour amongst Western Australian gay and bisexual male youth'. Health project submitted as part of the School of Health promotion, Curtain University, WA, Australia.

Don't Take Your Life Project (1998) (in progress). Primary Health Care Advancement Funded Project, Department of Human Services, South Australia, Australia.

Erickson, E. (1950) *Childhood and Society*, Norton, New York.

Faulkner, A. H. and Cranston, K. (1998) 'Correlates of same sexual behaviour in a random sample of Massachusetts high school students', *American Journal of Public Health*, 88 (2) pp. 262-266.

Garofalo, R., Wolf, R. C., Kessel, S., Palfrey, J. and Durant, R. H. (1998) 'The association between health risk behaviours and sexual orientation among a school based sample of adolescents', *Pediatrics*, 101 (5) pp. 895-902.

Gibson, P. (1989) 'Gay and lesbian youth suicide', in M.Feinlieb, (ed) *Prevention and Intervention in Youth Suicide, Report of the Secretary's Task Force on Youth Suicide*, Vol 111, pp. 109-142, US Department of Health and Human Services, Washington, DC.

Glover, S., Burns, J., Butler, H., Patton, G. (1998) 'Social environments and the wellbeing of young people' *Family Matters*, No 49. Autumn.

Goggin, R. and Sotiropoulos, T. (1994) *Sex in silence: a National study of young gays*, Australian Federation of AIDS Organisations.

Hammelman, T. L. (1993) 'Gay and Lesbian Youth: Contributing factors to serious attempts or considerations of suicide', *Journal of Gay and Lesbian Psychotherapy* 2(1), pp. 77-89.

Here for Life: Youth Suicide Prevention Forum (1998) August 10th-11th, Canberra, Australia.

Here for Life: Youth Sexuality Project (1996) Western Australia, http://www.queer.org.au/~wayouth/sponsors.html

Kourany, R. F. C. (1987) 'Suicide among homosexual adolescents', *Journal of Homosexuality*, 13 (4) pp. 111-117.

Kruks, G. (1991) 'Gay and Lesbian homeless/street youth; special issues and concerns', *Journal of adolescent health*, 12, pp. 515-518.

Kus, R. J. (1980) *Gay freedom: an ethnography of coming out*, PHD Thesis, University of Montana, DAI Vol 42-02A, p. 864, 423 pages.

La Barbara, P. (1994) *The gay youth suicide myth. The Lambda Report on Homosexuality. Telling the Truth Project*, Leadership U. http://www.vitualcity.com/youthsuicide/usdh.htm#2030

Millard, J. (1995) 'Suicide and suicide attempts in the lesbian and gay community', *Australian and New Zealand Journal of Mental Health Nursing*, 4, pp. 181-189.

Moscicki, E. K. (1995) 'Epidemiology of suicidal behaviours', *Suicide and Life Threatening Behaviour*, 25 (1), pp. 22-35.

Muehrer, P. (1995) 'Suicide and sexual orientation: a critical summary of recent research and directions for future research', *Suicide and Life Threatening Behaviour*, 25, *Supplement*, pp. 72-81.

National Health Medical Research Council (1997) *Depression in young people; Clinical Practice Guidelines*, National Health and Medical Research Council, AGPS, Canberra. Australia.

Olson, E. D., King, C. A. (1995) 'Gay and lesbian self –identification: A response to Rotheram-Borus and Fernandez', *Suicide and Life Threatening Behaviour*, 25, *Supplement*, pp. 35-39.

Ottawa Charter for Health Promotion (1986) An International Conference on health promotion. World Health Organsisation, Health and Welfare Canada. Canadian Public Health Association. Canada.

Proctor, C. D. and Groze, V. K. (1994) 'Risk factors for suicide among gay, lesbian and bi-sexual youths', *Social Work*, 39. Number 5. September.

Remafedi, G.(1987a) 'Adolescent Homosexuality; Psychosocial and medical implications', *Pediatrics*, 79, pp. 331-337.

Remafedi, G., Farrow, J.A., Deisher, R. W. (1991) 'Risk factors for attempted suicide in gay and bisexual youth', *Pediatrics*, 87 (6) pp. 869-875.

Remafedi, G., French, S., Story, M., Resnick, M. D. and Blum, R. (1998) 'The relationship between suicide risk and sexual orientation: results of a population based study', *American Journal of Public Health*, 88 (1), pp. 56-60.

Report of working party examining the purchasing of Mental Health Services for young gay, lesbian and bi-sexual people (1997) South Australian Health Commission, South Australia.

Rotheram-Borus, M.J. and Fernandez, M. I. (1995) 'Sexual orientation and developmental challenges experienced by gay and lesbian youth', *Suicide and Life Threatening Behaviour*, 25, *Supplement*, pp. 26-34.

Shaffer, D., Gould, M. S., Fisher, P., Trautman, P., Moreau, D., Kleinman, M. and Flory, M. (1996) 'Psychiatric diagnosis in child and adolescent suicide', *Archives of General Psychiatry*, 53, pp.339-348.

Shaffer, D., Fisher, P., Hicks, R. H., Parides, M., and Gould, M. (1995) Sexual orientation in adolescents who attempt suicide', *Suicide and Life Threatening Behaviour*, 25, *Supplement*, pp. 64-71.

Thatcher, M. (1987) Tory Party Conference. Cited in Equality 2000. Supplement to Gay Times.Issue 236, pp. 16-18 May.

Tremblay P. (1996) Health and Human Services, CDC, Youth Suicidality, pp. 1-16, http://www.virtualcity.com/youthsuicide/usdh.htm#2030

Uribe, V. and Harbech, K. (1992) 'Addressing the needs of lesbian, gay and bi-sexual youth: Project 10 and school based intervention', *Journal of Homosexuality* 24, pp. 9-28.

Walsh, J., Hillier, L. (1997) What Turns You On? Project, Cited in the National AIDS Bulletin. Australia.

Youth Risk Behaviour Survey, Seattle, WA. (1996) Safe Schools Anti Violence Documentation Project, 3rd annual report, Autumn. http:// www.vitualcity.com/ youthsuicide/usdh.htm#2030

Youth Risk Behaviour Survey, Vermount (1995) http:// www.vitualcity.com/ youthsuicide/usdh.htm#2030

Youth Risk Behaviour Survey, Massachusetts (1995) http:// www.vitualcity.com/ youthsuicide/usdh.htm#2030

Youth Suicide in Australia: The National Youth Suicide Prevention Strategy (1997) Commonwealth Department of Health and Family Services, Australian Government Publishing Service, Canberra.

6 Weaving the Threads of Mental Health Promotion in South Australia

ADRIAN BOOTH AND ANGELA BURFORD

Abstract

Mental health promotion is a relatively new, evolving and very exciting area of public health. The challenge for mental health promotion within Australia is 'weaving its many threads' through the various areas of mental health policy, programs and service delivery.

Working towards a definition of mental health promotion and supporting its approach has been hindered in Australia by the fact that such work has taken place within the context of mental health systems that have traditionally relied on curative, clinical and risk factor approaches to mental health issues and problems. Therefore mental health intervention has commonly been associated with mental illness at an individual risk level rather than that of addressing people's capacity across the population and developing supportive environments toward social and emotional well-being (Wood and Wise, 1997).

Despite these challenges mental health promotion has increasingly been receiving greater attention across Australia due to the necessity to promote the overall emotional and social well-being of the population. Reasons for this shift in thinking include the prediction that as we move toward 2020 depression will be the biggest health problem in the developing world and the second biggest cause of disease burden world-wide (World Health Organisation 1996). Increasing evidence of the efficacy and effectiveness of programs that promote mental health and prevent mental health problems and disorders has also influenced a move toward mental health promotion within the mental health system (Raphael, 1993; Scanlon et al, 1998; Tilford et al, 1997; Hodgson and Abbassi, 1995).

This paper will look at the current challenges that exist for mental health promotion within South Australia. These challenges are many in number however for the purposes of this paper the following areas have been chosen under the broad heading of moving beyond rhetoric to reality- translating the talk into action. developing a clear mental health promotion State-wide Framework ensuring consumers of mental health services are actively involved in the development of mental health promotion at a policy and/or program level convincing others to implement mental health promotion.

This paper will also highlight the importance of taking the opportunity to integrate mental health promotion as part of State-wide mental health initiatives.

Setting the Scene for Mental Health Promotion in South Australia

Currently in Australia there is a growing emphasis on the importance of undertaking a preventative or an early intervention approach. In 1992 the National Mental Health Strategy was agreed to by all State and Territory Health Ministers in Australia. The Strategy included the National Mental Health Plan (1992), the National Mental Health Policy (1992) and the consumer focused Mental Health Statement of Rights and Responsibilities (1991). This provided the opportunity in Australia to have a National Strategy to support people who have mental health needs. The vision of the National Mental Health Strategy has been to:

- promote the mental health of the Australian community and, where possible, prevent the development of mental health problems and mental disorders;
- reduce the impact of mental disorders on individuals, families and the community;
- assure the rights of people with mental disorders.

Currently a second National Mental Health Plan which renews the Strategy to 2001 is with the Health Ministers of the States and Territories of Australia for endorsement. This second plan mirrors the increased attention to promote mental health, prevent mental health disorders and reduce the overall burden associated with mental health disorders and problems on individuals, families, communities and the health and welfare system.

Since 1992, in South Australia a period of reform within the Mental Health Service has taken place. Some significant changes have resulted in:

- increased access for consumers and carers through the process of

regionalisation of mental health services;
- improved service quality;
- increased awareness and acceptance of mental health and mental illness in the community;
- improved information about the way mental health services are delivered.

In 1995 a realignment process began which aimed to devolve the centralised South Australian Mental Health Service to regional local responsibility.

In December 1997, following a coronial review of the State Mental Health Service the Minister for Human Services initiated a Mental Health Summit which led to a 'community based consultation' which provided South Australia with a context to examine what strengths,weaknesses, gaps and priorities exist for the mental health system.

As a consequence of the community consultations and workshops a five point plan has been developed which involves:

- a commitment to increase mental health funding over the next five years;
- development of services which are targeted to meet the needs of particular groups across AS;
- a development framework for education and training for both health workers and consumers and carers;
- developing community support networks;
- an injection of capital funds to ensure the regionalisation process continues (Brown, 1998).

As a consequence of the Mental Health Summit a South Australian Mental Health Strategic Plan is being developed to help guide and incorporate the 5 point plan.

Mental Health Promotion in South Australia

In 1993 the Mental Health Promotion Program was established as part of the Health Promotion Unit, Public and Environmental Health Service. Its role is to provide leadership and promote opportunities to implement mental health promotion activity across South Australia.

Leadership for mental health promotion has also been undertaken by different groups and individuals, paid and unpaid, trained and untrained and from government and non government sectors in South Australia. Consequently mental health promotion programs and projects have been undertaken across the life stages (infancy through to older persons) and across various settings (home, workplace and schools). Such activity demonstrates the remarkable contribution that people, both inside and outside of the 'health system' (for example, self help and community groups) across South Australia, have made to other people's mental health and social and emotional well-being.

A number of definitions for mental health have been developed. Raphael (1993) states that the important attributes of good mental health are:

> ... happiness, competence, a sense of power over one's life and positive feelings of self esteem...as are the capacities to love, work and play.

Another definition that has been proposed is:

> Mental health is the emotional and spiritual resilience which enables us to enjoy life and survive pain, disappointment and sadness. It is a positive sense of well being and an underlying belief in our own and others' dignity and worth (Health Education Authority, UK, p. 7, 1997).

These definitions begin to challenge the notion that mental health is only about illness or sickness. Achieving good mental health is related to a complex interplay of physical, social, cultural, environmental, economic and spiritual factors. Our mental health is constantly influenced by these factors and also by what has been termed throughout the literature as protective or risk factors. Protective factors can be:

- having strong friendships or support;
- being employed;
- feeling a sense of connection with one's surroundings;
- living in a safe, secure environment.

Risk factors that can lead to poor mental health can be:

- being unemployed;
- feeling powerless and/or isolated;
- being marginalised;
- being in a violent or abusive environment.

In defining mental health promotion it can be argued that it covers everything that leads to ensuring and maintaining positive mental health for the whole population and segments within it. Given this broader viewpoint, mental health has been described as:

> the capacity of individuals and groups to interact with one another and the environment in ways that promote subjective well-being, optimal development and the use of cognitive, affective and relational abilities and the achievement of collective goals consistent with justice (Mental Health-Statement of Rights and Responsibilities, Canberra, 1991).

There are many threads to mental health promotion. Currently in South Australia a State paper is being prepared to compliment the work already undertaken in South Australia but, more importantly to provide a context to describe and support its future (Booth and Burford, 1998).

Evidence now strongly supports the effectiveness of mental health promotion programs. Work undertaken in the United Kingdom has noted that there are benefits in using a mental health promotion approach. They are:

- promoting mental health may reduce the incidence or severity of mental health problems;
- morally, society has a responsibility to advocate and undertake mental health promotion in fostering good mental as well as physical well-being;
- promoting good mental health leads to individuals adopting meaningful and effective roles in society (Health Education Authority, UK, p 2, 1997).

Similarly there has been other work which has been done on the overall effectiveness of mental health promotion intervention (Hodgson and Abbassi, 1995; Trent and Herron, 1997;Tilford et al, 1997).

Historically much of the activity in mental health promotion has taken place without any formalised definition of what mental health promotion is and has therefore lacked an integrated framework which could guide its theory, practice and overall measurement of effectiveness.

The many threads of mental health promotion that have been identified as part of literature reviews, mental health program development and individual practitioner experience are listed below:

- providing and developing a working definition of mental health promotion;
- identifying mental health protective and risk factors;
- describing mental health promotion theory and practice;
- developing mental health promotion indicators and agreed outcomes;

- measuring the effectiveness of and evaluating mental health promotion intervention;
- exploring and formulating funding options for mental health promotion activity;
- identifying roles and responsibilities for individuals who work within or outside of the health sector;
- developing a mental health promotion framework which supports and guides activity.

In order that mental health promotion is successfully woven throughout a mental health system all these components need to be addressed.

Challenges for Weaving the Threads of Mental Health Promotion in South Australia

The South Australian Mental Health Summit has provided the chance to review priorities for the mental health needs of the South Australian population. With the establishment of the 5 point plan (Brown, 1998) for mental health services in South Australia and the development of a State-wide Strategic Plan there is the opportunity to 'weave the threads' of mental health promotion through the fabric of the South Australian mental health system and other health and non health sectors. Critical to achieving this step is to move beyond rhetoric to reality; in other words, translate the talk into action.

1. Developing a Clear Mental Health Promotion State-wide Framework

Mental health promotion can be diverse in nature and varied in approach. Given the complex interplay between social and physical environments and individual health status the development of a mental health promotion framework is vital in reducing risk factors that impact on an individual's or population's social and emotional well-being. Utilising a framework approach has also assisted in developing mental health promotion priority areas as part of the South Australian State-wide Mental Health Strategic Plan. The Ottawa Charter (1986) is widely used in South Australia as a framework to address the complex and multi-faceted nature of promoting and maintaining health.

The Ottawa Charter states that the achievement of good health outcomes will most likely occur as the result of collaborative effort and co-operation between various organisations, agencies, services and groups across the health and non-health sector. In South Australia we have seen people and organisations working together to address many specific mental health issues. These include homelessness, violence, women and depression, transcultural mental health issues and Child and Youth health. The following five action areas of the Ottawa Charter provides an excellent framework for continued mental health promotion activity in South Australia:-

Building healthy public policy Mental health promotion needs to be integrated into the design of policy across all sectors at all levels including schools, workplaces, hospitals and community based organisations. The integration of mental health promotion as part of the development of the South Australian Mental Health Strategic Plan is a current example of how mental health promotion can be 'woven' into State planning and Regional mental health service delivery.

Creating supportive environments Emotional resilience, citizenship and developing healthy structures (Health Education Authority, UK, p 7, 1997) are integral components of how individuals cope with day to day life issues and how they interact with other people. These three themes are also involved in the creation of supportive environments which include settings such as the workplace, the family, school and the community. Feeling safe, supported and being recognised as a valued citizen of society all influence a person's mental health.

Strengthening community action There has been a strategic shift to involve and develop partnerships with consumers, carers and young people within South Australia. This has been prompted recognising consumers of mental health services as active participants in reviewing mental health services across South Australia. The South Australian Mental Health Summit represented a significant milestone in encouraging this shift toward community involvement.

Developing personal skills Included in the five point plan is the need to develop a framework around education and training for the professional workforce and carers and consumers within South Australia. Developing personal skills leads to improved knowledge, attitudes and beliefs toward mental health issues. Some examples of personal skill development include a Partnership with Young People Project which involves working with young people on mental health issues and a volunteer led companion project which aims to decrease isolation within a country community.

Re-orientating health services toward prevention South Australia has started to recognise that its mental health service needs to reorientate towards early intervention and prevention in addition to providing clinical and curative based services. This means that clinical services are undertaken within a wellness as opposed to an illness setting. The 'Weaving The Threads of Mental Health Promotion' South Australian State Paper (Booth and Burford, 1998) will provide the context for informing and enhancing the knowledge base of what mental health promotion is and what its various 'threads' consist of.

A Conceptual Framework for developing initiatives in mental health promotion has been undertaken within New South Wales, Australia, which has utilised the five action areas of the Ottawa Charter across a health care and mental health status continuum (Scanlon and Williams, 1997).

2. Ensuring Consumers of Mental Health Services are Actively Involved in the Development of Mental Health Promotion at a Policy and/or Program Level

Developing respectful and trusting partnerships with consumers, carers and young people has been an increasing focus of the South Australian Mental Health Service. Supporting the co-ordination of a consumer run State Conference entitled "Our Lives Our Choices" and utilising the arts in promoting consumers' experiences of mental illness forms part of the current mental health promotion activities across South Australia.

Respectful practice has been the foundation which has assisted in developing partnerships with young people. South Australia is recognised nationally as a leader in promoting partnerships with young people. Some examples of respectful practice involve including young people as part of State mental health Committees and developing supportive environments based on mutual learning and respect.

3. Convincing Others to Implement Mental Health Promotion

Although there has been an increasing shift toward undertaking a mental health promotion approach across Australia, there are still barriers to overcome. Some of these include:- uncertainty regarding exactly what mental health promotion is, differing opinions on appropriate outcome measures, the uncertainty regarding the difference between prevention and promotion, lack of experience and confidence in working in mental health promotion, funding options for mental health promotion activity. Work towards setting outcomes for mental health promotion has been undertaken (Wood and Wise, 1997; Kickbush, 1996) and increased attention has been given to developing evidence based programs that modify risk or protective factors for mental health problems and/or disorders (Mrazek and Haggerty, 1994; Raphael,1993). Future work in these and other areas such as population based surveys having wellness in addition to sickness indicators included are vital in enabling us to build on our knowledge of what maintains people's well-being.

Conclusion

Weaving a mental health promotion garment for South Australia depends on a number of issues, for example - is our cotton (language) compatible? - is the design of the garment (Mental Health State Plan/Mental Health Promotion State Paper) jointly owned and recognised by all those making it? - is the use of the garment sustainable over time or will it slowly disintegrate?

Our belief is that we can weave positive,empowering threads of mental health promotion throughout our States mental health system (garment) however we will need to ensure that all the threads of mental health promotion as highlighted in Table 1 are part of the 'weaving' activity. In addition it is important that we learn from research which builds on our knowledge of outcomes for and evaluation of mental health promotion so that our garment remains intact and an inspiration to all that look at it.

References

Booth, A., and Burford, A. (1998) Mental Health Promotion in South Australia - Current issues and future directions. Department of Human Services (paper in progress), South Australia.

Brown, Hon. D., MP, Minister for Human Services, South Australia (1998). Speech given to the Mental Health Summit on Wednesday 6th May. Adelaide, South Australia.

Hodgson, R., and Abbassi, T. (1995) 'Effective mental health promotion. Literature review', *Technical Reports No 13,* Hybu Lechyd Cymru Health Promotion Wales, Cardiff, Wales.

Kickbush, I. (1996) 'Setting Health Objectives: The Health Promotion Challenge', Keynote address presented to the Healthy people 2000 Consortium meeting "Building the Prevention Agenda for 2010: Lessons learned", New York.

Mental Health Promotion: A Quality Framework (1997) Health Education Authority, London.

Mental Health Statement of Rights and Responsibilities (1991) Report of the Mental Health Consumer Outcomes Task Force, Australian Government Publishing Service, Canberra.

Mrazek, P., Haggerty, R. (eds) (1994) *Reducing risks for mental disorders. Frontiers for preventative intervention research,* National Academy Press, Washington.

National Mental Health Plan (1992) Commonwealth Department of Health and Family Services, Canberra.

National Mental Health Policy (1992) Australian Health Ministers, Australian Government Publishing Service, Canberra.

Ottawa Charter for Health Promotion (1986) An International Conference on health promotion, World Health Organisation, Health and Welfare Canada, Canadian Public Health Association, Canada.

Raphael, B. (1993) *Scope for prevention in mental health,* National Health and Medical Research Council. Commonwealth of Australia.

Scanlon, K., Williams, M. and Raphael B. (1998) 'Mental health promotion in NSW. Conceptual framework for developing initiatives', *NSW Public Health Bulletin,* Vol 9 No 4, pps. 43-46, State Health Publication 98-0043.

Scanlon, K. and Williams, M. (1997) *Mental Health Promotion in NSW. Conceptual framework for developing initiative,* NSW Mental Health Service.

Tilford, S., Delany, F. and Vogels, M. (1997) *Effectiveness of mental health promotion interventions. A review,* Number 4 in the Health Promotion effectiveness reviews, Health Education Authority, London.

Trent, D. and Herron, S. (1997) 'Sharing the way to success: The value of model programs', *Paper presented at the Mental Health Promotion Conference in Maastricht.*

Wood, C. and Wise, M. (1997) *Building Australia's capacity to promote mental health: Review of infrastructure for promoting mental health in Australia,* National Mental Health Strategy: Working Together for Mental Health.

World Health Organisation (1996) *Report of the Ad Hoc Committee on Health Research and Development,* World Health Organisation, Geneva.

7 Social Integration and Mental Health Promotion

ODD STEFFEN DALGARD

Abstract

Mental health promotion initiatives may be targeted towards different social units e g. a local community or neighbourhood. It is then of crucial importance to identify those stressors which adversely impinge up mental health if we are to develop effective promotion/prevention programmes.

Social disintegration i.e. the fragmentation of social networks, apathy, lack of social interaction and leadership and feelings of powerlessness and pessimism is conducive to a state of poor mental health. Social disintegration may have a number of causes including rapid social change, high migration rates, poor economic conditions and cultural/social conflicts but whatever the individual causes we need to acknowledge their inter-dependence and cumulative effect.

This paper describes three projects which illustrate how social disintegration contributed to poor mental health in different communities and then discusses how effective interventions were implemented to bring about improved mental health status in the populations under review.

Examples 1 and 2, the Stirling County and the Eastlake studies are based upon mental health promotion intervention programmes. The third project relates to the analyses of the development of the social environment in different neighbourhoods in Oslo. This is not an intervention project but a study that discusses how mental health may be improved when the social environment itself is subject to improvement - 'a delayed community development'.

The special nature of these programmes is that they combine features of the community development with epidemiological research, thus making it possible to assess the effect of social change on mental health, in terms of the level of change in the prevalence of mental health problems. Such validation is essential if mental health initiatives are to be stringently evaluated.

The Stirling County Study

This widely acknowledged study took place in Nova Scotia in the 60s under the guidance of Alexander Leighton and colleagues (Leighton 1965, Leighton & Murphy 1985). The initial stage of the study was purely epidemiological and investigated the relationship between social disintegration and mental health problems, mainly in terms of depression and anxiety.

Social problems within the County meant that a number of communities were characterised by high levels of unemployment, fragmented social networks, lack of local leadership, weak social organisations and levels of anxiety and depression, which were noticeably in excess of those found in well integrated communities.

One of the 'deprived' communities 'The Road' was selected as the subject for a community development programme.

The aims of the programme included increasing:

a) social integration through improved patterns of social support and mutual aid
b) cognitive assets by increased educational opportunities and
c) economic resources.

Through the combined effort of the education authorities, the use of community development techniques and improvements to the economic environment the three aims of the project were successfully addressed within 'The Road' community.

It is important to emphasise the importance of the role played by the inhabitants of 'The Road' who took an active role in the development process by establishing a number of initiatives including community clubs and co-operative organisations. The programme organisers acted as advisers and provided information but did not accept a formal leadership position.

A second survey, which followed some ten years later, illustrated the standard of living in 'The Road' had improved and there was a rise in the levels of education. Other features of change noted were that many adults were now in semi-skilled jobs and there was a growth of business ventures created by the pooling of capital; a more co-operative approach being evident with increased awareness of individual responsibility. Of great significance was the reduction in the prevalence of mental disorders which moved to the same level as that of the rest of Stirling County.

The Eastlake Study

The Eastlake Study, described in Mental Health and the Built Environment (Halpern 1995), was carried out in a housing estate of 712 dwellings constructed some twenty years previously.

The initial survey indicated a poor functioning neighbourhood suffering from a number of symptoms associated with social disintegration e g. the majority of residents were young families with children and a relatively low income, there was a high degree of isolation and relatively high levels of anxiety and depression.

Over a period of two years the estate was subjected to a refurbishment programme with a special emphasis on safety and security. New traffic regulations were brought in, there was improved lighting, a scheme to strengthen windows, enclosure of gardens, the closure of alleyways and a general improvement in landscaping.

The project, conducted by a team from Cambridge University, actively encouraged resident participation throughout the whole process.

At the follow-up stage, which took place about 12 months after the intervention, there were significant changes in the physical environment and to both the social environment and the mental health of residents. For example there was greater social interaction and people were more trusting of each other. The feelings of pessimism and uncertainty changed to become more optimistic with a belief in the future and people on the estate felt a stronger identification with the neighbourhood (eg whereas only 22 per cent described Eastlake as good or very good for children to grow up in at the beginning this changed to 52 per cent at the follow-up stage).

Halpern emphasised increased interaction between people and the enhanced feeling of neighbourhood cohesion as being very important for the improvement of mental health.

Oslo Study

The third example is based on my own research, analysing the development of the social environment and states of mental health in different neighbourhoods in Oslo. Hence this is not an intervention project, but rather a study which describes how mental health may improve when the social environment improves as part of a normal development process. The reason for including this study in a paper about mental health promotion, is that the knowledge gathered by the study may contribute to the formulation of certain guidelines for the planning of new neighbourhoods conducive to good mental health.

The study started about 15 years ago with a major epidemiological survey in Oslo conducted by myself, that looked into the prevalence of mental disorders in different types of neighbourhoods *(Dalgard 1986)*. Some 1000 randomly picked people from 5 major types of neighbourhoods were interviewed according to a structured questionnaire, measuring mental health in the same way as *Leighton* had done in Stirling County. Ten years later a follow-up, using the same questionnaire as in the initial study was undertaken. I then reinterviewed 503 people still living in Oslo or surrounding communities.

In the initial study, significant variations in rates of mental disorders between difference neighbourhoods were found. The highest prevalence was found in a new "satellite town" in the outskirts of the city, characterised by a relative lack of public and private services, few recreational opportunities, economic problems, high migration and qualitatively poor social networks. This difference in mental health status could not be explained away by differences in the socio-demographic background of people, as the pattern did not change much when controlling for a number of socio-demographic factors in a multivariate statistical analysis (MCA).

It appeared likely that the high prevalence of mental disorders in this areas *(area V)* was at least partly caused by a social environment that combined low social support with various stressors, e.g economic problems, lack of recreational opportunities and a poor environment for children to grow up. However, it was difficult to rule out the possible effect of social selection, even if one tried retrospectively to control peoples mental health before moving into their present neighbourhood.

In the following I will focus especially on the people who continued to live in the same neighbourhood during the follow-up period, allowing for intra-pair comparison of mental health and related psycho-social variable between T1 and T2 (T1 -original study &T2-follow up) and relate this to changes in the neighbourhood. The description of the neighbourhoods was partly based on the respondents own assessment at the two points in time, partly on data from key informants.

One methodological problem related to this approach, was that the sample studied was substantially reduced, and that selective migration could influence the results. The possibility obviously existed that people who continued to live in the same neighbourhood were a special selection with respect to mental health and related psychosocial variables, and for this reason interpretation might be difficult. Another possibility, that also would make interpretation difficult, was that people who objected to taking part in the follow-up interview could also represent a special selection. To allow for this, as far as possible, people who had moved, or people who had refused to take part in the follow-up, were compared with the rest with respect to psychiatric and psycho-social characteristics at T1. To summarise there did not seem to be strong selection effects associated with moving or non-participation at T2. The final sample was fairly representative with respect to sex, marital status, social support and most important, mental health at T1. With this in mind we can look at some of the results.

In the following we will compare the development in *area* V with the development in the other areas taken together. The number of people followed in *area V* was 31 compared with 233 in the other areas *(Dalgard & Tambs 1997)*.

Discussion

As shown in *Figure 1* there was a significant improvement of mental health in *area V,* whereas there was not change with respect to mental health in the other areas.

With respect to social support the trend goes in the same direction, with more improvement in *area V* than in the other neighbourhoods. This trend however is not statistically significant.

If the improvement of mental health in *area V* was caused by improvement in the environment, one should expect more change for the better in *area V* than in the other neighbourhoods. Both objectively and as perceived by the respondents this was the case. With respect to change in neighbourhood quality, as described by key informants from the social welfare offices, there was a substantial improvement in *area V,* whereas there had been no change in the other areas. For example in *area V* a new school had been commissioned, play grounds for children were extended, a sports arena and park were built, more activities for adolescents were organised, a shopping centre with restaurant and cinema was opened and the subway line was extended to the neighbourhood.

In conjunction with the above the assessment of the respondents also showed a positive change. This is illustrated in *Figures 2-6. In Figures 2, 3 and*

Figure 1: Psychiatric Symptoms at T1 and T2 by Area of Living: Non-Movers

Mean score

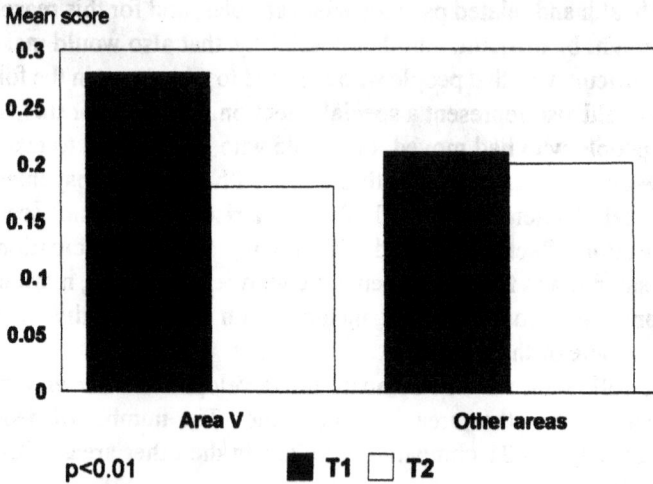

p<0.01 ■ T1 □ T2

Figure 2: General Evaluation of the Neighbourhood by Area of Living: Non-Movers

Percent content

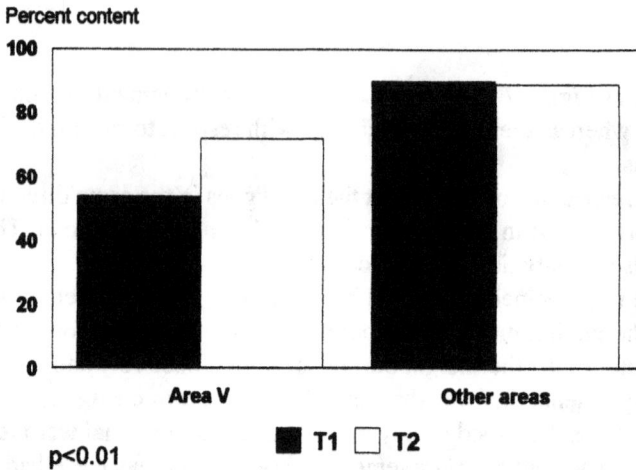

p<0.01 ■ T1 □ T2

4, which compares the situation at T1 and T2 in *area V* with the general assessment in other areas, we can see there is a substantial improvement in *area V* particularly in respect of the environment for children and adolescents.

Figures 5 and 6 show there has been no significant changes in the other areas.

Although the findings indicate the positive effect of an improved social environment on the mental health status or residents there are a number of

Figure 3: Evaluation of the Neighbourhood: Area V, Non-Movers

Percent content

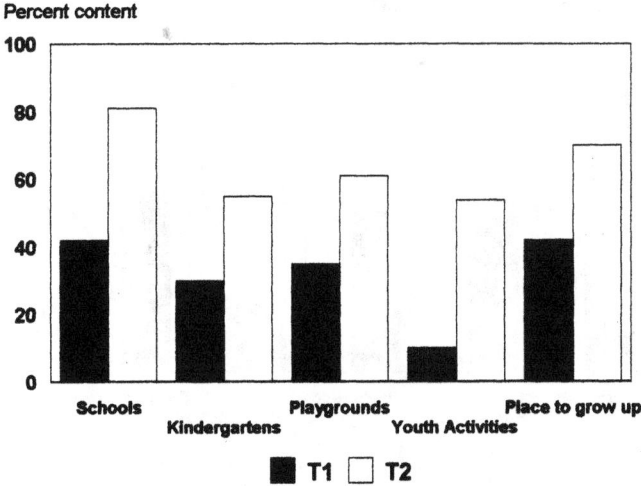

Figure 4: Evaluation of the Neighbourhood: Area V, Non-Movers

Percent content

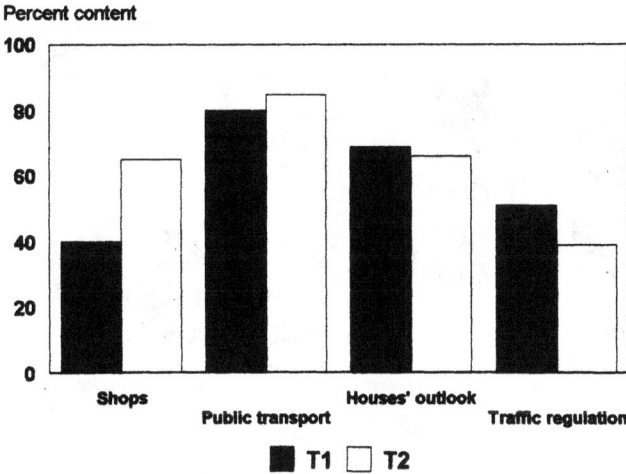

issues we must consider in interpreting the findings. For example improvements of the mental health of the residents in *area V* may simply reflect a better adaptation to the environment during the follow-up period, irrespective of what might have happened in terms of environmental changes. As *area V* was a relatively new housing development, i.e. some 8 years old, with a high level of new residents this 'better' adaptation effect may have been especially strong with the neighbourhood, thereby explaining why the residents mental health had improved more than in other areas. One method of

Figure 5: Evaluation of the Neighbourhool: Other Areas, Non-Movers

Percent content

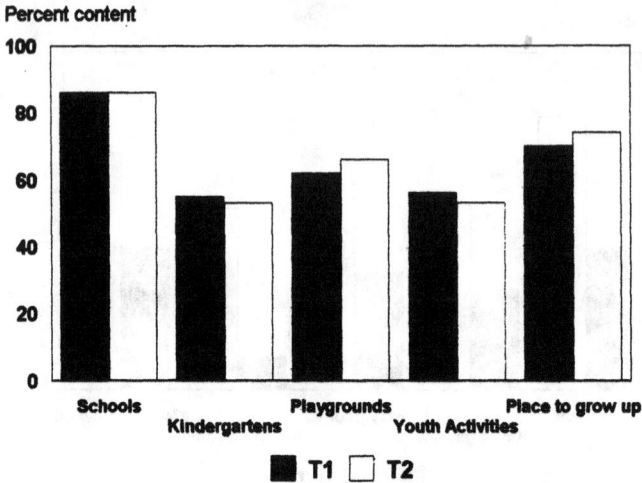

Figure 6: Evaluation of the Neighbourhood: Other Areas, Non-Movers

Percent content

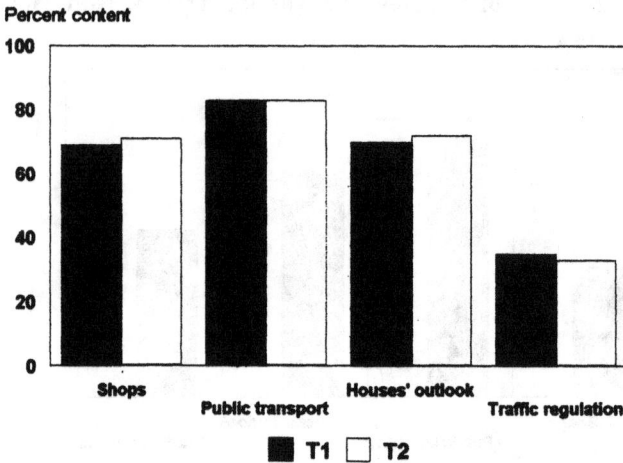

control is to take the statistical analysis of the length of stay in the neighbourhood at Ti into consideration. When doing this in a multivariate statistical analysis, where a number of socio-demographic variables were included, there was still a significant effect on the mental health status of those living in area V. Hence the positive change in the social environment does appear to correlate with an improved mental health status.

Conclusion

From a preventative position the present study does give rise to some optimism even if there is still some way to go in respect of moving from theory to practice in this complex field. The findings of the study indicate that the selection of residents on the grounds of their social status, in combination with the poor provision of social and other recreational facilities, especially for young families with children, led to a negative effect on the mental health of residents in *area*. More effective planning would more probably reduced levels of mental distress. In reality the 'appropriate' neighbourhood facilities e g social, recreation etc were only put into place between the dates of the first study and the follow up research some ten years after the neighbourhood was built. This delay could well have hindered the social integration of the neighbourhood and as a consequence reduced the quality of life in *area V* and led to an increased prevalence of mental disorders.

To prevent the occurrence of the type of social and psychological problems described in *area V* a set of guidelines for the planning of new neighbourhoods, taking into account the findings from this and other epidemiological studies, has been formulated and published by *The National Institute of Public Health (1997) in Norway*. The guidelines (see below) can be used for example by the municipal health services in their efforts to offer advice in their matters concerning the community's mental health and it's promotion.

Guidelines for the Planning of New Neighbourhoods

- develop the housing areas in stages;
- arrange for the necessary public and private services before people move in;
- vary the age composition;
- avoid concentrating people with special problems in certain blocks;
- build neighbourhoods of limited («human») size;
- vary the type of housing, allowing for a multigenerational community;
- provide special houses or flats for collective activities and social interaction;
- establish recreation areas for different age groups;
- promote neighbourhood organizations responsible for various social activities;
- encourage future inhabitants to participate in planning of new neighbourhoods.

References

Dalgard, O. S. (1986) 'Living Conditions, Social Network and Mental Health', in S-O Isacsson and L. Janzon (eds) *Social Support - Health and Disease*, Akmquist and Wiksell, Stokholm.

Dalgard, O. S. and Tambs, K. (1977) 'Urban environment and mental health A longitudinal study', *The British. Journal of Psychiatry, 171,* 530-536.

Dalgard, O. S. *(1977) Noermiljo og psykisk helse Mentalhygieniske retningslinjer for planlegging av mye bomilijoer,* Folkehelsa, Oslo.

Halpern, D. (1995) *Mental Health and the Built Environment,* Taylor and Francis, London.

Leighton, A. H. (1965) 'Poverty and Social Change', *Scientific American* 212, 21-27.

Leighton, A. H. and Murphy, J. M. (1985) 'Primary prevention of psychiatric disorders' in O. S. Dalgard (ed) *Preventive psychiatry - methods and experiences*, Acta Psychiat. Scand no. 337, vol. 76.

8 Enhancing Parenting Skills

DR. KEDAR NATH DWIVEDI

Parenting must be one of the most important tasks that any sentient being performs. Societies or cultures become altruistic or narcissistic through the processes of parenting.

> Luckily a great deal of parenting just happens naturally Also good or bad parenting has a tendency to breed itself. A piece of iron, for example, by being in contact with a magnet, becomes magnetised and in turn can magnetise another piece of iron. Similarly the qualities of parenting tend to get transmitted and flow like a river *(Dwivedi, 1997a:1-2)*.

Parenting is a bit like

> pottery, where there is a need for balance between the hand inside and the hand outside the clay on the wheel. Similarly in parenting, one hand is concerned with intimate emotional care, support and nurturing while the other hand sets boundaries, promotes better emotional and behavioural management and offers discipline. Without the hand inside, the pot is likely to break. In the absence of the hand outside, it can assume a form that is very ugly *(Dwivedi, 1 997a; 2)*.

By being in touch with the fantasies, feelings and needs of the child within, one is able to get in touch with the fantasies, feelings and needs of the child without. Parenting is thus built upon the foundation of empathy. It is like developing a taste for delight in the delight of others. And it is also very natural as one often sees a baby being delighted in the delight of the parent and the parent being delighted in the delight of the baby.

Luckily, parenting is rightly attracting more political attention now. There is already an All-Party Parliamentary Group for Parenting in the UK a Parenting Forum exists to highlight and campaign for parenting education. There is also a proposal to create an Institute of Family and introduce Parenting Order to deal with delinquency.

There is an intimate relationship between Parenting and Mental Health as both influence each other. It is not only the mental health of children but also of parents that is affected by parenting and affects parenting in turn. Mental disorders in the child can easily produce a strain on parenting. Conflict between parents, mental health problems in parents and other children and even family breakdowns can occur. Similarly a number of parental mental and personality disorders can seriously affect parenting process. Good and bad parenting contribute to child's mental health and mental disorder respectively. Feelings of belonging and of confidence, good self esteem, communication and emotional management skills require good parenting. Various emotional, conduct and other mental disorders in children (for example, anxiety, depression, enuresis, drug and alcohol abuse, self harm, eating disorder and so on) tend to be contributed by parenting problems. Children with mental disorders are more likely to have mental health problems in their adulthood along with an impact on their own parenting. Similarly for parents, the experience of good parenting helps with their self worth and emotional well being.

Parenting enhancement programmes have an important place within each aspect of a comprehensive mental health service, such as, rehabilitative, curative, preventive and promotive services. In addition to secondary prevention, parenting has a significant role to play in primary prevention of mental and personality disorders. It has also been argued that secondary prevention (that is, a high-risk approach) may be the preferred way where the epidemiological distribution is of bimodal nature such as, in blood sugar. However, in situations where the epidemiological distribution is of a continuous nature, such as, childhood behaviour problems, the most effective way of tackling this is not by secondary prevention but by primary prevention or population approaches (Stewart Brown 1998).

Parenting programmes are often designed to utilise group work principles. Groups can be classified in many different ways. Some of these classifications are as follows.

- Open; slow open; closed; drop-in
- Structured vs. spontaneous/unfolding
- Heterogeneous vs. homogenous
- Homogenous may be according to
  Parents'

Age	e.g. young parents, learning disability;
Circumstances	e.g. step parents; foster parents; adoptive parents; single parents; gay parents;
Issues	e.g. child abuse, post-natal depression; drug abuse; bonding, expectations.

Children's
      Age   e.g. Pippin, Newpin, Adolescents.
      Issues/disorders   e.g. ADHD; Anorexia; Dyslexia, Drug
                             abuse; Bullying, Conduct Disorder (Parenting
                             Orders); encopresis; epilepsy, self-esteem;
                             home work, learning disability and so on.

There are a variety of approaches that can be adopted in initiating parenting programmes. Some of these are as follows.

1. Establishment of Self help groups, mutual support groups, clubs, associations and so on. For example, a school in Northamptonshire organised a study day on parenting for the parents of the children attending the school. Towards the end of the day a parents association for this purpose was formed which has continued to organise activities for enhancing their parenting skills.

2. Educational programmes. There are several examples of such programmes which aim to educate parents in relation to various parenting tasks (such as, Protective Behaviour), childhood problems (such as, Attention Deficit Hyperactivity Disorder, Anorexia, Drug abuse, Autism etc.) or issues (such as, self esteem).

3. Psycho-educational programmes aim to clarify principles, which are ten applied to individual circumstances as a part of the programme. Use of adult education principles and indirect approaches, such as, narrative and stories can be very useful (Dwivedi, 1997b). Some examples of psycho-educational programmes are as follows.

- Systematic Training in Effective Parenting or STEP (Dinkmeyer et al 1997)
- Behaviour Management
  NCH Action for Sick Children: Handling Children's Behaviour Project
  Fun with the Families (in Leicester)
- Cognitive approaches
  To deal with expectations, attributions, problem solving, anger and stress management (Stern & Azar, 1998).
- Webster-Stratton Programme (Webster-Stratton, in press).

4. Group analytic group work (Behr, 1997). This is an experiential approach, which moves at the pace of the parents. They are helped to learn by exploring the connections between the relationships within the group

with their experience as parents to their children and of relationships in connection with the way they themselves were parented.

5. Interactive programmes are based upon training parents as they interact with their children in relation to various parenting activities, such as, Feeding; Home work; Play and so on (Dwivedi, et al 1994, Foote et al, 1998).

6. Programmes to help a Meta perspective. These are programmes that create an opportunity for the parents to obtain a Meta perspective on their parenting and improve matters as they see fit. Videotaping of parent child interactions and playing this back to them usually does this. It can also be combined wit group work (Marsden-Allen, 1997).

Parenting Programmes can be developed through a variety of agencies and channels. Some examples are as follows:

- School curricula and preparation for parenthood
- Media
- Reaching parents through
- Schools (e.g. Adult education activities and programmes designed around children's educational issues)
- Social Services, such as, in relation to child protection, children in need and the recent emphasis on refocusing.
- Police, such as, in relation to Drug abuse, delinquency, Parenting Order.
- Health, such as, in relation to mental disorders in children (Hyperactivity, Conduct Disorder and so on) and in parents (Post-natal Depression)
- Voluntary Agencies, such as, Home-Start, Newpin, Pippin and so on.

In addition to local initiatives, there is a need for galvanising more national and international initiatives. National initiatives can arise not only through the governmental organisations but also through the voluntary sector. Thus, the proposed Institute of Family, national curricula, Young Minds, Parenting Forum and other organisations can play an enormous role in such initiatives. Similarly international initiatives can come from a variety of channels, such as, through International Child Development Centre, National Childbirth Trust, La Leche, Save The Children Fund, UNICEF, UNESCO, Inclusion International, International Initiative, The Clifford Beers Foundation and others.

There is also an urgent need to evaluate the effectiveness of various parenting programmes and their specificity. The review by Barlow (1997) and Stewart-Brown (1998) are valuable steps in that direction.

References

Barlow, J. (1997) *Systematic Review of the effectiveness of parent-training programmes in improving behaviour problems in children aged 3-10 years,* Health Services Research Unit, Oxford.

Behr, H. (1997) 'Group Work with Parents', in K. N. Dwivedi (ed) *Enhancing Parenting Skills.* Chichester, John Wiley & Sons.

Bornstein, MIT-I (ed) (1995) *Handbook of Parenting.* (vols 1-4) Erlsbaum Associates, Mahwah, NJ.

Dinkmeyer, D., McKay, G. D. and Dinkmeyer, D. (1997) *The Parents Handbook* (STEP), Circle Pines, American Guidance services.

Dwivedi, K.N. (ed) (1997a) *Enhancing Parenting Skill,* John Wiley & Sons, Chichester.

Dwivedi, K.N. (1997b) *Therapeutic Use of Stories*, Routledge, London.

Dwivedi, K. N., Lovett, S. B., Jones, M H., Wright, J. M. and Woolley, E. (1984) 'Family Treatment on a Day Treatment Basis: a Case Illustration'. *A.F.T. Newsletter,* August: pp. 3-9.

Foote, R.C., Schuhmann, E. M., Jones, M. L., & Eyberg, S.M. (1998) 'Parent-Child Interaction Therapy: A Guide for Clinicians', *Clinical Child Psychology and Psychiatry.*3(3): pp. 361-373.

Marsden-Allen, P. (1997) 'Developing Home-based Parenting Skill Programmes, supported by group sessions of parenting techniques', in K. N. Dwivedi (ed) *Enhancing Parenting Skills,* John Wiley & Sons, Chichester.

Stewart-Brown, S. (1998) 'Evidence based child mental health promotion: the role of parenting programmes', in K.N. Dwivedi (ed) *Evidence Based Child Mental Health Care,* Northampton Child and Adolescent Mental Health Service.

Stern, S. B., & Mar, S.T. (1998) Integrating cognitive strategies into behavioural Treatment for Abusive parents and Families with Aggressive Adolescents. *Clinical Child Psychology and Psychiatry.* 3(3): pp. 387-3403.

Webster-Stratton (in press) 'Preventing conduct disorder in the Head start: Strengthening Parenting Competencies in Children', *Journal of Consulting and Clinical Psychology.*

9 From the Margins to the Mainstream: the Public Health Potential of Mental Health Promotion – or Mental Health Promotion – what works?

LYNNE FRIEDLI

Mental health is the emotional and spiritual resilence which enables us to enjoy life and to survive pain, disappointment and sadness. It is a positive sense of well-being and an underlying belief in our own, and others' dignity and worth.[1]

Introduction

In this paper, I would like to briefly outline the case for building a new agenda for mental health promotion, drawing on the growing literature on social capital, as a rationale for placing mental health at the centre of a new public health debate. I will then go on to discuss what we know about effectiveness and conclude with a brief reference to themes of the World Mental Health Day Campaign for 1998.

A wide range of new public health initiatives in the UK, including Health Action Zones, Health Improvement Programmes, Primary Care Groups and Healthy Living Centres, provide a framework for integrating mental health promotion and strengthening both formal and informal support for mental health. Current government policy on social inclusion, employment, housing and transport highlight the importance of thinking beyond traditional service boundaries – they also provide an opportunity for putting mental health on a wide range of agendas. While it is now generally recognised that health is largely determined by socio-economic factors, the word 'mental' is rarely heard in these contexts. On the contrary, there is a prevailing myth that mental illness is something which affects a small number of people and that the issue is only of concern when public safety is threatened. A more radical agenda might begin by recognising that everyone has mental health needs, whether or not they have a diagnosis, and make explicit the centrality of mental health to all areas of policy.

What is Mental Health Promotion?

Mental health promotion is essentially about promoting the capacity for mental health at three levels:

- strengthening individuals or increasing emotional resilience;
- strengthening communities;
- reducing structural barriers to mental health.[2]

Strengthening individuals includes increasing emotional resilience, through interventions designed to promote self-esteem, life and coping skills, communicating, negotiating, relationship and parenting skills. It also includes promoting resourcefulness, through developing skills to improve the capacity to cope with life events, transitions and stresses e.g. parenting, bereavement, redundancy or retirement.

Strengthening communities includes initiatives to increase levels of social inclusion and participation and the capacity of communities to tackle issues which affect mental health e.g. anti-bullying strategies, afterschool childcare schemes, family friendly policies in the workplace, community safety, and supporting and facilitating social and self-help networks.[3]

Reducing structural barriers to mental health may involve policy and partnership initiatives to reduce inequality and discrimination and to promote access to meaningful occupation, adequate housing, appropriate services, equal opportunities and, for example, reductions in alcohol and drug misuse.

Another approach is to see mental health promotion as a kind of immunisation, working to increase the resilience of individuals, organisations and communities – as well as to reduce conditions which are known to damage mental well-being in everyone, whether or not they currently have a mental health problem.

There is, of course, an extensive literature on protective and risk factors for what I have called emotional resilience and a wide range of interventions which seek to increase the self esteem, coping, and lifeskills of individuals.[4] Current debates about social capital provide a unique opportunity to begin to address more systematically the other levels – strengthening communities and reducing structural barriers to mental health.

Social Capital

Social capital, like mental health, is a resource which benefits individuals but can only be developed in relationship with others. Putnam, Kawachi, Wilkinson[5] and others have identified indicators of social capital in terms of trust, tolerance and reciprocity, or levels of civic engagement and association – essentially the strength of the social fabric – as opposed to a 'neighbourhood of strangers'. And there is a growing body of research which suggests that the strength of social capital, the structure of relations between people, is as important as personal resources in determining life chances.[6]

Richard Wilkinson, in his influential book, 'Unhealthy Societies', makes a compelling case for the link between inequality and health.[7] Income distribution, the size of the gap between rich and poor, is clearly related to mortality rates in all the major causes of death, including alcohol related, accidents, homicide, crime, violence and drug use. These latter causes are of course significant because of clear links between, for example, abuse of alcohol and emotional and psychological problems.

The importance of this for a mental health agenda, is evidence of the link between inequality and the decline of social capital, or the disintegration of the social fabric. Wilkinson argues that psycho-social burdens are now the most important limitation on the quality of life – citing eight reviews showing strong links between social integration and mortality.[8]

The significance of social networks and social support in maintaining health, particularly in the face of life events/transitions like bereavement, has long been recognised.[9] At a wider, community level, the strength of the social fabric is associated with positive health and helps to limit the damaging impact of economic deprivation or other causes of trauma. How people feel about themselves and others, and their relationship to the broader community (over and above any personal or family networks) may be a key determinant of health. In a cross sectional ecologic study based on data from 39 states, Kawachi et al found that lower levels of social trust were associated with higher rates of most major causes of death, including coronary heart disease, malignant neoplasms, cerebrovascular disease, unintentional injury and suicide.[10] Repairing the social fabric, from this perspective, will require a recognition of the centrality of social, psychological and emotional deprivation. As Wilkinson observes:

to feel depressed, cheated, bitter, desperate, vulnerable, frightened, angry, worried about debts or job and housing insecurity; to feel devalued, useless, helpless, uncared for, hopeless, isolated, anxious, a failure: these feelings can dominate people's whole experience of life... It is the chronic stress arising from feelings like these which does the damange. It is the social feelings which matter, not exposure to a supposedly toxic material environment.[11]

Wilkinson's argument, of course, is that it is inequality, the gap between rich and poor, which creates the exclusion giving rise to these stressors. From our point of view, what is equally significant is the evidence of the impact of psycho-social factors on overall health.

Mental health promotion has a crucial role to play in reducing and limiting the impact of psycho-social stressors, both through strengthening individuals and through strengthening and supporting a diversity of social, communication and information networks, which link people within the community. These include self-help, advocacy, neighbourhood and voluntary activities, as well as structures which facilitate community planning and local decision making in the provision of services.[12] The key words here are **access** (to services in the widest sense), **participation** (in planning and implementation) and **influence** (over the decision making process).

In this vision, meeting mental health needs depends on a society characterised by high levels of civic engagement and explicit recognition of the impact of public policy and practice, in all sectors, on mental health.

Effectiveness and Mental Health Promotion

So how does what we know about effectiveness fit in here? There is a growing literature on effectiveness and although there is a need for more research, there is sufficient evidence to justify investment in a wide range of interventions.

Effective interventions fall into three broad categories:

- changing knowledge, attitudes and awareness;
- enhancing life skills;
- strengthening social support.

Campaigns

Campaigns or mass media interventions, particularly if supported by local community action, can have a measurable impact on knowledge, attitudes and behavioral intentions.[13] Campaigns which focus on advocacy techniques, for example generating unpaid publicity in the press or setting the news agenda through creating positive mental health stories, can also play a proven role in influencing opinion formers and the climate of public opinion.[14] Mass media interventions can be used successfully:

- to increase understanding of mental health problems;
- to reduce stigma;
- to increase knowledge of how to cope and sources of help and support.

Strengthening Individuals

There is now a substantial literature demonstrating the effectiveness of a range of interventions which aim to reduce symptoms of mental distress and increase or strengthen individual resilience.[15] These include:

- cognitive behavioural therapy;
- brief interventions (alcohol);
- life/social skills;
- parenting skills;
- exercise;
- art.

Two examples are of particular interest:

Prescription for leisure There are now nine studies of randomized control trials showing the value of exercise in reducing mild symptoms of depression and anxiety, and promoting better GHQ scores.[16] Aerobic exercise is as effective as cognitive therapy in reducing depression and anxiety and less costly. The beneficial effects are not dependent upon the intensity of the exercise i.e. walking is as effective as jogging, moderate exercise as effective as intense exercise. Evaluation of 'Balance for Life' in Essex found that the ten week programme of exercise significantly reduced depression and anxiety, increased overall quality of life and self-efficacy for exercise. 68% of clinically depressed patients had depression scores that became non-clinical within three months.[17]

Arts on Prescription Arts on Prescription provides access to art and creative activities including poetry, painting, music and pottery. Arts on Prescription can be combined with Prescription for Leisure, allowing entry to a range of activities for people experiencing mild to moderate depression. There is some evidence that arts activity for former psychiatric in-patients results in fewer readmissions.[18] Evaluation of the Arts on Prescription project in Stockport showed an improvement in GHQ scores, better self-concept, an increase in social activities and less use of other services.[19] The Kings Fund has developed an evaluation framework suitable for arts based health work, which was pioneered in partnership with 'Looking Well' an arts based community project in North Yorkshire.[20]

Strengthening Communities

Effective interventions include the following:

Self-help and social support Referral to self help groups is as effective as cognitive therapy and medication in treating generalised anxiety disorders and active participation in user groups has a wide range of benefits.[21] With the formation of Primary Care Groups, there is a good case for rethinking primary care boundaries, expanding the role of pharmacists and primary care nurses, for example, and creating meaningful links between social, voluntary and informal care and support. Primary care also has the potential to provide a referral and support service to increase awareness of and access to existing sources of support within the community, including self-help, advocacy, user groups, voluntary agencies, as well as creative, leisure, sporting and educational facilities. The internet has considerable potential as a resource, greatly extending access to lay and informal sources of support and information. The new technology can extend the reach of the Primary Health Care Team and, perhaps more significantly, build on and reinforce different communities' own resources and capacities.

Anti-bullying schemes The Olweus study in Norway showed that being a bully or a victim of bullying at school is a predictor for later problems, including conduct disorders, crime, and alcohol abuse (bullies) and depression, anxiety and suicidal behaviour (victims). There is therefore a strong case for including anti-bullying strategies as a key mental health promotion intervention. These should include zero tolerance for bullying – every child has a right to be safe at school, a period of consultation which enables parents, teachers, school governors and the wider community to sign up to the principles of anti-bullying, and clearly understood strategies for reporting and acting on bullying incidents.[22] Similar initiatives should also form part of a broader mental health promotion policy within the workplace.

Health at work There is evidence that work factors are not just associated with ill health, but actually cause it. Positive working conditions can protect people in vulnerable situations, for example increased control at work and greater social support reduce the stress associated with a high workload. The Nuffield review, based on Cochrane criteria, concluded that systemic, organisational programmes supported by a mixture of staff and management training were most effective, including the following (all of which have implications for mental health):[23]

- training skills, notably around problem solving and decision making;
- communications skills training;
- interpersonal awareness;
- organisational stress management;
- exercise.

Key characteristics of mentally health promoting workplace:

- workload appropriate to capabilities of individual;
- opportunities to control pace of work;
- clear, fair performance appraisal, feedback, development/training opportunities;
- equal opportunities and understood guidelines on sexual and racial harrassment and bullying;
- personal responsibility and recognition;
- home/work balance;
- security and safety;
- consultation, communication, opportunities for involvement;
- good social support.

Measuring Success

Having outlined some of the approaches to mental health which are effective, I want to conclude with some thoughts on potential indicators.

Indicators: Process

Mental health promotion process indicators can be summarised under the following headings:

- access;
- inclusion;
- participation;
- influence;
- integration;
- impact.

The basic principles of service provision in all sectors (local authorities, health authorities and trusts, voluntary agencies and the private sector) can themselves be process indicators for mental health promotion - notably in relation to access, inclusion, user/client involvement, clarity about how decisions are made, seamless provision and cultural sensitivity. Within the mental health field, attention has rightly focussed on mental health service user experiences of services and developing approaches to improve these at all levels. However, there is also a need to look more broadly at the mental health impact of a wide range of services, including schools, the criminal justice system, housing, residential care and transport, particularly in relation to differential access and the exclusion of particular groups or communities.

In addition, some measure of integration, for example links between or evidence of routes to informal, alternative or complementary approaches could provide a valuable measure of progress towards seamless care and effective partnership across the voluntary/professional divide.

Indicators: Outcome

Building on what I have described in relation to social capital, there is considerable potential for beginning to develop indicators which are measures of mental well-being, rather than relying solely on measures of mental illness or the presence or absence of symptoms. These include:

- general well-being;
- feeling safe;
- feeling connected (i.e. people round here generally look out for each other);

- participating;
- feeling involved (i.e. able to influence decisions which affect my life);
- days lost to mental health problems (quality of life);
- knowledge of positive steps (what to do when down/unable to cope;
- action on postive steps (have taken action to look after my mental well-being);
- mental health promotion policies.

WMHD Campaign 1998

Finally, I want to describe briefly the themes of the WMHD Campaign, which is funded by the Department of Health and co-ordinated in England by the HEA. The campaign focus this year is on challenging discrimination as a positive step for mental health, looking specifically at the experiences of four groups who are particularly likely to experience discrimination:

- older people;
- mental health service users;
- black and Minority Ethnic Groups;
- Lesbians and Gay men.

Focussing on discrimination provides a framework to:

- highlight the discrimination faced by mental health service users;
- address the dual discrimination faced by users who are gay or older or from Black and Minority Ethnic Groups;
- move mental health up the agenda in organisations and communities concerned with racism, homophobia and ageism;
- increase understanding of the damaging impact of discrimination on mental health.

Discrimination remains a central isue for anyone who has, or will have, a mental health problem. Discrimination is also a mental health issue for all those who experience exclusion – and, as I hope I have shown, there is growing evidence that exclusion damages not only those who are excluded, but the whole community, with an impact on the health and well-being of everyone.

Notes

1 Health Education Authority *Community Action for Mental Health* 1998.
2 Further discussion of definitions of mental health promotion in *Mental Health Promotion: A Quality Framework* HEA 1997 p.7-11.
3 Examples of community based initiatives are included in HEA *Community action for Mental Health* 1988.
4 Effective interventions in areas like parenting skills, pre-school education, life skills etc are cited in *Mental Health Promotion: A Quality Framework* HEA 1997.
5 Robert Putnam *Making Democracy Work: Civic Traditions in Modern Italy*, Princeton, 1993; Richard Wilkinson *Unhealthy Societies: The Afflictions of Inequality* London 1996; Paul Hoggett et al *Urban Regeneration and Mental Health in London: A Research Review* University of West of England & Centre for Mental Health Services Development, London 1997.
6 Two key reports suggest the significance of social capital for current debates: The Commission on Wealth Creation and Social Cohesion *Report on wealth creation and social cohesion in a free society* London, 1995; Report of the Commission on social Justice *Social justice: strategies for national renewal* London, 1994; see also the Demos Report by Leadbiter, *Social Entrepreneurs*; links between unemployment and mental distress have been related as much to exclusion from social networks as to material deprivation cf Kammerling and O'Connor 'Unemployment rate as a predictor of psychiatric admission' *British Medical Journal 307* p1536-1539, 1993; Wilkinson cites reports by Rosengren and Whelan which demonstrate the crucial importance of social support in reducing mortality associated with stressful life events cf Rosengren et al 'Stressful life events, social support and mortality in men born in 1933' *British Medical Journal 307*, p1102-5, 1993; Whelan 'The role of social support in mediating the psychological consequences of economic stress' *Sociology of Health and Illness 15* p.86-101 1993; In a study of deprived children in the USA, Runyan et al found that the presence of indicators for social capital increased developmental thriving by up to 66% see Runyan DK et al 'Children who prosper in unfavourable environments: the relationship to social capital' *Paediatrics 101* p.12-18 1998.
7 Wilkinson 1996 ibid.
8 Berkman 'The role of social relations in health promotion' *Psychosomatic Research no 57* p. 245-254 1995; Berkman cites 8 community studies between 1979 and 1994 which show an assocaition between social integration and mortality – i.e. people who are isolated are at increased mortality risk from a number of causes. Kawachi makes a similar point using USA data. Donnelly et al *Opening New Doors* HMSO, London 1994; Hoggett 'What is Community Mental Health' *Journal of Interprofessional Care No 7,3*, 1993; Hoggett (ed) *Contested Communities* Bristol, 1997.
9 The classic text is Brown & Harris *The Social Origins of Depression* 1978; see also Donnelly ibid; on the impact of racism see Christie & Smith 'Mental Health and its Impact on Britain's black Community' *Mental Health Review 12,3* p.5-14,

1997: between 1988 and 1992 the level of reported racist attacks increased by more than 75%. Wilkinson cites a range of studies which highlight the impact of the way in which work is organised on health – lack of control, communication, and job insecurity.

10 Kawachi 1997.

11 Wilkinson p.215.

12 Bloom B.L., *Life event theory and research: implications for primary prevention* Washington 1985 provides a thorough review of research on factors which mitigate stressful life events, with social support and social networks identified as crucial.

13 Barker C, Pistrang N et al 'You in Mind, a preventive mental health television series' *British Journal of Clinical Psychology* 1993 p281-293; Sogaard AJ & Fonnebo V 'The Norwegian Mental Health Campaign in 1992: part 2: changes in knowledge and attitudes *Health Education Research 10* p 267-278; Hersey JC, Klibanoff LS et al 'Promoting social support: the impact of California's "friends can be good medicine" campaign' *Health Education Quarterly 11(3)* p.293-311 1984.

14 Hastings, Stead, Whitehead et al 'Using the media to tackle the health divide: future directions' *Social Marketing Quarterly* 1998 in press.

15 see for example Hosman C, Veltman N *Prevention in Mental Health: A review of the effectiveness of health education and promotion* Utrecht 1994; HEA 1997 ibid; Hodgson RJ & Abbasi T *Effective Mental Health Promotion: literature review Health Promotion* Wales 1995 Cardiff.

16 Glenister D 'Exercise and Mental Health: a review' *Journal of the Royal Society of Health* p.7-13 January 1996.

17 Darbishire L and Glenister D *The Balance for Life Scheme: Mental Health Benefits of GP recommended exercise in relation to depression and anxiety* Essex 1998; see also a write up of this case study in *Community Action for Mental Health* HEA 1998.

18 Colgan et al *START* in Huxley P *Arts on Prescription: an evaluation* 1997; see also Phillip R and Robertson I 'Poetry helps Healing' *The Lancet 347* 1996; a case study of exercise and arts on prescription in Stockport is included in *Community Action on Mental Health* HEA 1998.

19 Huxley ibid.

20 Angus J and Murray F *Evaluation Frameworks, Criteria and Methods in Arts-for-health* Kings Fund 1996; Winn-Owen J 'The declaration of Windsor' *The role of humanities in medicine, arts, health and wellbeing; beyond the millenium* Nuffield Trust 1998.

21 Tyrer et al *The Lancet* 1988; Barnes & Shardlow 'From passive recipient to active citizen: participation in mental health user groups' *Journal of Mental Health 6,3* p289-300 1997; Stark W 'Empowerment and Self-help initiatives – enhancing the quality of psychosocial care' in Jenkins and Ustun (eds) *Preventing Mental Illness: Mental Health Promotion in Primary Care* p 291 –297 1998.

22 Olweus Dan *Bullying at school: what we know and what we can do* Blackwell, London 1993.

23 Nuffield Report *Improving the Health of the NHS Workforce: Report of the Partnership on the Health of the NHS Workforce* 1998; see also Borrill CS, Wall TD, West MA et al 'Mental Health of the workforce in NHS Trusts' Universities of Sheffield and Leeds, March 1996 – ongoing research; Health Education Authority *Working for your health: a survey of NHS Trust Staff* 1997; Health Education Authority *Fit to face the future? Maintaining a healthy workforce for the NHS* 1998; Doherty N and Tyson S *Mental well-being in the workplace: a resource pack for management training and development* Health & Safety Executive 1998.

10 Three Aspects of Mental Health Promotion in the Department of Mental Health Rome E

ALESSANDRO GRISPINI AND RENATO PICCIONE

Abstract

The Department of Mental Health (DSM) Rome E is one of the Italian Institutions which try to promote the achievement of preventive measures in the mental health field.

The three following areas represent the priorities: 1) the development of the "social enterprise", 2) the de-institutionalisation process in all structures of the department and in particularly in the Diurnal Centres, 3) engagement of adolescents.

1. The "social enterprise" is the locus of integration, work and cooperation in which therapists, suitable patients, professional figures of working world try to create a productive activity that competes in the working market. This is quite different from the classic concept of "ergotherapy", a procedure well known in psychiatric hospitals. The "social enterprise" represents the opportunity for patients to produce goods and services that have a real existance and that have a real remuneration, something very close to real life. The "social enterprise" creates the opportunity for the social matrix to absorb what - the mental illness- was in past rejected and this, ultimately, modifies the social representation of patients in the general population.

2. The continuous de-institutionalisation process implies three interdependent and complementary aspects: a) giving up the net of asylum (avoiding reproducing it in community care), b) creation of supportive net in the community to improve the opportunity for patients to achieve relationship and human rights, c) promotion of different way of thinking towards mental illness.

3. The DSM Rome E provides a service for adolescents which carries out systematic integration with 30 high schools of our District.

Italian psychiatric culture deems that prevention doesn't exist and it is a pure chimerical project. More consideration is given to mental health promotion which is the first level of preventive paradigma (Mrazek and Haggerty, 1994).

What do Italian Departments do to Carry Out and Empower Mental Health Promotion Strategies?

In a recent national congress we organized on the issue "Prevention and Mental Health" (Rome, 1997) we discovered with pleasure and surprise that several initiatives were carried out throughout every part of Italy. These initiatives were lacking in organization and did not have a real integration with other aspects of daily activities.

Despite the fact that public psychiatric services in Italy are named "Department of Mental Health" their main purpose is to treat severely disturbed patients by rehabilitative and specific psychotherapeutic treatments. Less severe patients are also treated with psychopharmacological and psychotherapeutic approach, but almost all financial and structural resources are devoted to severe patients, above all chronic schizophrenic ones.

The Department of Mental Health Rome E for a resident population of 570.000 has 8 Centres of Mental Health, 2 psychiatric wards for acute patients (24 beds), 5 Diurnal Centres, 4 Therapeutic Communities, 2 Accommodation Communities, 14 apartments, 1 unit for adolescents, 1 unit for prevention, an evaluation group.

Those working in these structures number 370, to a large extent psychiatrists, psychologists, social workers and nurses. Therapists of psychodynamic, systemic and sociological background are in the main. The number of cognitive therapists is gradually increasing. Psychiatrists with a strict biological training are few. Almost all the therapists adopt mixed model.

Patients undergoing treatment in 1997 numbered about 6,000. This number increases each year about 10% and this creates considerable problems among the therapists.

Several Italian Departments are considerably articulated and can offer specialized treatments for the different types of mental disorders, but very few Departments try to encourage a preventive culture in the different aspects of daily activities.

The Department of Mental Health Rome E has been involved for years in trying to change this state of things. We have several good reasons to improve the preventive interventions in Italian services, but we are far from accomplishing this goal even in our Department.

As Mrazek and Haggerty (1994) pointed out, *mental health promotion measures* are the very first step in preventive work. They are called *"universal"* because the main target is not the illness but the maintenance of mental health in general population. These type of interventions should be without risk and at a low costs.

Despite the fact that the Italian Departments show an unsatisfactory attitude for prevention, we believe that Italian model for psychiatric care represents a strong and powerful resource for promotion of mental health.

How does the Italian Model of Psychiatric Assistance Work to Improve Mental Health?

The cornerstone of the Italian model rests on the concept of *de-institutionalisation* which is often confused with that of de-hospitalisation. The de-institutionalisation process implies three interdependent and complementary aspects: 1) giving up the "safety net" of the asylum (avoiding reproducing it in community care), 2) creation of supportive net in the community to improve the opportunity for patients to achieve relationship and rights, 3) promotion of different way of thinking towards mental illness.

The de-institutionalisation process means: a) the continuous overcoming process of pathological dependence of psychiatric patients from any kind of psychiatric institutions and b) the avoiding of the vicious circle illness/pathological responses towards illness (Saraceno, 1995, p. 6).

This process has been developing with, at the beginnig, a breakdown in accademic culture and later in continued involving powerful conflicts.

I will focus my presentation on the way the three aspects I mentioned before are carried out in the Department of Mental Health Rome E. In particular, I am going briefly to describe the following three issues: 1) the development of "social enterprise", 2) the continuous de-institutionalisation process of our structures, looking carefully at with Diurnal Centre, 3) mental health measures for adolescents and the general population.

The De-institutionalisation Process and "Social Enterprise"

One of the most important meanings of de-institutionalisation process is to create social and relationship opportunities for patients. This goal counteracts the well known lack of social relationships (and human rights) which we may observe in severe patients. Franco Basaglia, the leader of the Italian movement that brought down psychiatric hospitals, used to say that we should "put in brackets" the illness and deal with the person and his/her problems. From this point of view, taking care of the patient it is not simply a technical matter, but the re-creation of a relationship process. This can not be achieved only with a technical measures, split from the social body. Basaglia and his followers stressed the role of non professional operators in the recontruction of relational field. This statement encountered strong resistances in academic psychiatry.

Nowadays, the role of technical interventions is full accepted even amongst Basaglia's most orthodox followers even, but at the same time the core of his teaching is also accepted in wide sectors of academic psychiatry. The old quarrel is fading away. One of the most important achievement of Basaglia's original teaching is what we call "social enterprise". What do we mean by this concept and how does it work in promoting mental health in the community?

Social enterprise is the locus of integration, work and cooperation in which psychiatric therapists, patients, professional figures of the working world try to create a productive activity that competes in the market. This is quite different from the classic concept of "ergotherapy", a procedure well known in psychiatric hospitals. The latter was a real exploitation inside an isolated context. The social enterprise represents the opportunity for patients to produce goods and services that have a real existence and that have a real remuneration, something very close to real life.

We can not, in this context, outline the theoretical foundations of social enterprise (De Leonardis et al.,1994; Saraceno, 1995). We are trying here to argue that social enterprise creates the opportunity for the social matrix to absorb what - the mental illness- was in the past rejected. The very close cooperation between the ill and the non-ill modifies the social representation of mental illness. And this, ultimately, carries out the de-institutionalisation process that represents the inescapable step - not alone of course- for mental health promotion. From this point of view, the de-institutionalisation process and the social enterprise mean the increasing of protective factors.

De-institutionalisation Process in Community Centres

In our model a good quality of integration amongst different therapeutic and rehabilitative community centres can be a risk factor or a protective factor for the mental health of people who live in the community. Yet Italian Departments of Mental Health are not safe from the risk to reproduce a pathological functioning. When the therapeutic community, for example, admits patients without a clear project for the long term or when the main problem for a therapist is to find a "bed" for his/her patient, we are dangerously approaching an out-of-date way to meet people's needs.

We could put forward similar arguments for Centres of Mental Health which should represent the propulsive core of therapeutic projects for patients and the source of initiatives for looking after the mental health of the general population. Too often we must ascertain that these centres work as specialist centres with operators who work as they were in private office and not as a team.

We would like to say a few words on Diurnal Centres. Amongst several therapeutic and social activities (psychotherapic, expressive, entertainment, summer and week-end holidays) our Diurnal centres - jointly with private cooperatives - are trying to develop- experiences of social enterprise: 1) promotion of training and working opportunities for patients, 2) creation of green areas for the general population inside one of the most over-crowed and neglected neighbourhoods of Rome, 3) setting up catering services for the residential structures of the Department, 4) restoration laboratories, 5) biological agriculture, 6) production of decorated glass windows.

These activities are not "entertainment", but productive work with public and private purchasers. They involve public and private staff, the most suitable patients, wide sectors of general population, volunteers, public institutions, all cooperating to achieve social and productive aims, partially supported by public resources, but partially sustained by their profits.

In our Department a specific team has been made up to coordinate and develop different social enterprise experiences. The main goal is to achieve a strong social enterprise, competitive in the working market, which produces training and working opportunities for patients as well as a new culture of mental health in the community.

Mental Health Promotion for Adolescents

The third contribution of our Department for mental health promotion is the creation of a specific service for adolescents. The quality of the Italian public services for adolescents is very low. We do not have yet a proper department for childhood and adolescence. All problems concerning the young people are under the domain of so called the "Mother-Infant Department" which is not equipped enough to treat the psychological and neuropsychiatric problems. Our Department is the only one in Italy which has carried out a specific service for young people aged from 16 to 23.

The aim of this service is equally devoted to improve mental health promotion measures and treat mental disorders.

The former task is accomplished through establishing strong relationships with the thirty high schools of our community.

The main goals are: a) to give opportunities to "enrich normality" in adolescents by encouraging the ability to establish relationships and expanding social network for themselves and their families, b) to improve self - coping attitudes, c) to increase a better representation of public services for mental health (reducing the stigma and feelings of shame to be needed for help), d) to reduce scholastic drop-outs, e) to increase interactive abilities of teachers, enabling them to detect mental states at risk.

We have three main tools to intervene in the school (Piccione, Grispini,1998): 1) psycho-educational programs for students, families and teachers; 2) the continuous counselling process devoted to teachers and students; 3) the so called " class-group", in which all students of a specific class meet with a monitor, during ordinary school time, to discuss and explore freely several experiential and psychological problems (individuation-separation process vicissitudes, their life in family, their relationship with teachers and with the peer-group, general and specific problems of adolescence, self -coping attitudes, etc.).

References

De Leonardis O., Mauri D., Rotelli F. (1994), *L'impresa sociale*, Anabasi, Milano.
Mrazek P.J., Haggerty R.J. (Eds) (1994), *Reducing risks for mental disorders*, National Accademy Press, Washington, D.C.
Piccione R., Grispini A. (Eds) (1998), *Prevenzione e salute mentale*, Carocci Editore, Roma.
Saraceno B. (1995), *La fine dell'intrattenimento*, Etaslibri, Milano.

11 The State of the Art of Prevention in Italian Psychiatric Services

ALESSANDRO GRISPINI, RENATO PICCIONE AND
RENATO FRISANCO

Abstract

The Department of Mental Health (DSM) Rome E is actively involved in promoting preventive awareness among public psychiatric services.

In a recent survey which engaged about 800 centres we tried to explore
several issues: a) who is going to conduct prevention, b) by improving the
preventive paraigma, what will be the consequences for the Departments, c)
what are the most important strategies of prevention, d) what preventive activities can be planned and carried out, e) what are the most important hindrances that interfere in accomplishing preventive measures.

The most significant answers were the following five: 1) global lack of
trust, pessimism and sceptisism regarding operative possibilities in preventive
field, even by open - minded therapists, 2) promotional activities are considered realistic goals to be achieved, 3) almost all interviewees think that prevention and mental health promotion do not regard DSM only, but involve all
social health services, 4) the majority of the interviewees deems that prevention means promotion of mental health and only 1.7% think that the target has
to be the early detection and early treatment of mental conditions at risk, 5)
reducing of occurrence of new cases is considered a mere chimerical project.

Despite the fact that preventive culture in Italy is weak, there is strong
evidence that forces us to outline the need for implementation of preventive
model in the Departments. The four reasons for prevention are the following:
1) epidemiologic data, 2) the problem of *saturation* of psychiatric services, 3)
economic reasons and 4) clinic data.

The following four strategies are needed to improve psychiatric services: 1)
the managment of mental health is based on the community model and the con-

tinuous de-institutionalisation process, 2) the promotion of a new culture of mental health in school, 3) the introduction of brief, economic and effective therapeutic tools to treat non severe mental disorders, 4) early interventions in pre-psychotic phases and mental states at risk.

The issue of prevention and promotion of mental health is not well rooted and defined in Italian psychiatry. In a previous survey (Cozza, Napolitano,1996) on the quality of psychiatric services, the following six points arose.

1) Only two of 180 DSM put on preventive activities in their future programes.
2) Only 12.5% of the DSM have planned guidelines to establish links with General Practitioners.
3) Despite the fact that 46% of Italian DSM's carried out preventive and promotion of mental health activities, most of them lacked methodological coherence and were marginal.
4) The main aim of the DSM regards treatments and rehabilitative measures.
5) All the financial and human resources are completely devoted to treatment and rehabilitative techniques.
6) The theory of prevention and promotion of mental health was seen as weak and not well defined.

This is the background. The DSM RM E has been involved in a strong promotion of the preventive paradigma since 1986.

We have published 2 books on this issue (Piccione, 1994; Piccione, Grispini, 1998 a). We organized specific courses for operators of mental health and a national conference ("Prevention and Mental Health" held in Rome, 1997). One of the most important initiatives we have undertaken to increase the preventive practice in our Department is the opening of a service for adolescents. This service has established a strong relation with all highschools of our district. The main purpose has been the accomplishment of preventive programs for the mental health promotion that we described elsewhere (Piccione,Grispini,1998 a).

In 1997 we carried out a survey to further explore the state of the art of prevention in Italian psychiatric services.We sent to all psychiatrists/psychologists in charge of Italian Centres of Mental Health a questionnaire made up of 15 items that explored the following six issues:

1. Who is going to conduct prevention?
2. By improving the the preventive paradigma, what will be the consequences for the Department of Mental Health?

3. What are the most important strategies of prevention?
4. What preventive activities can be planned and carried out in your Department?
5. What are the most important hindrances that interfere in accomplishing preventive measures?
6. What initiatives have been carried out to improve the preventive culture and practice in your Department?

We delivered the questionnaire and we received 20% (149) of the initial sample (745) back. We are not going to describe in details all 15 items of the questionnaire and all multi-answers we received back from the Centres of Mental Health, but we will focus our presentation on five main points.

1. The Conductor of Prevention

Of the entire sample, 46% answered that prevention and mental health promotion do not regard DSM only, but involve all social-health services.
Of interviewees, 23% thought that the task of prevention has to do with the community in toto.

The others considered that the DSM is the principal resource for prevention.

2. The Consequences for DSM in Introducing the Preventive Paradigma

Of the interviewees, 60% think that improving the preventive culture will bring about a transformation of psychiatric services.
Forty seven per cent deemed that prevention has to become a priority and its achievement will promote the participation of family associations, volunteers, citizens, other formal and informal agencies.

Only 22.5% of the entire sample think that prevention will affect the style and quality of global interventions.

3. Strategies of Prevention

Prevention in psychiatry means, for the majority of the interviewees, promotion of mental health, in particular the psycho-education of the general population. Schools, public agencies, opinion leaders and so called " spreaders of information" are seen as the most available tools to promote a new culture based on preventive paradigma. Twenty six per cent think that prevention should be addressed to groups and working places at risk, but only 1.7% deem that the target has to be the early detection and early treatment of the mental conditions at risk.

This item shows, better than others, the state of the art of the preventive culture in Italian psychiatry. The culture of promotion of mental health is strong and well established owing to the particular Italian situation founded on the theory and practice of the de-institutionalisation; at the same time all preventive measures are identified with promotion activities and this brings about a weak model of prevention. Many Italian psychiatrists and psychologists, for example, still argue that early detection and early treatment in adolescents at risk for psychosis have to be avoided because of the risk of producing a new stigma.

4. What Preventive Measures can be Planned and Carried Out?

While the previous item has to do with the theoretical space of prevention, the 4th regards the practices that have actually been planned and are being carried out in Italian Departments. Beyond the different answers, the main fact is that Italian services are not able to plan effective preventive measures and the quality of the few initiatives carried out - above all educational activities for the general population- is unsatisfactory.

Rare is the relationship with general practitioners, with the exception of very few but remarkable services.

5. The Most Important Hindrances

The most reported answers are a) the lack of financial and human resources and b) the dominant paradigma based on the concept of " repairing damage". Other answers are: c) the lack of integration with other public agencies, d) the weakness of theoretical background, e) the lack of involvement of general society in mental health problems.

The Four Reasons for Prevention

Despite the fact that the preventive culture in Italy is weak, there is strong evidence that forces us to outline the need for implementation of preventive model in psychiatric culture and practices.

1. The first one derives from *epidemiological data*. As you know, about 20% of the general population suffers from some kind of mental distress. 15% have common emotional problems and 4% suffers from well-established mental disorders. It is obvious that the psychiatric services can not counteract all this mental suffering using merely therapeutic and rehabilitative interventions.
2. The second reason has to do with the problem that we call "*saturation*" of psychiatric services. Our data (Piccione et al.,1995) show that the number of patients under the care of the Departments of Mental Health rises by 10% every year, due to the increasing length of treatments for psychotic and non psychotic patients. In a few years the psychiatric services risk not being able to intake and manage the new help requests. The most severe patients and the neurotic patients and the widespread archipelago of those with common emotional disorders - some of whom at risk becoming severe patients - could be dismissed and, sometimes, abandoned. We need to develop more economic but effective instruments of intervention.
3. The third reason is *economic*. We do not intend describing in detail this technical problem, but we want to mention an aspect of it. Our Department receives the highest budget and has 5% of the total budget of the entire complex of health services that are in the District. The other Departments in Rome do not receive more than 2-3% of the budget. It is evident that this is a shortage of resources to devote to preventive and promotional activities which are, furthermore, difficult to evaluate and reimburse.
4. The last but certainly not less important reason for prevention is *clinic*. Many Authors pointed out that the delay between the onset of psychosis and the beginning of treatment results in a poor outcome. We need to implement models of intervention during the pre-morbid phase or in the early pre-psychotic phase (McGorry,1998).

Four Strategies to Improve the Psychiatric Services for the Next Decade

The strategies we are going to outline regard not only Italian Departments, but all psychiatric services that aspire to become modern organizations for the promotion of mental health and not remain as services that work only for "repairing damage".

1. *The managment of mental health is based on the community model and the continuous de-institutionalization process.* This means that psychiatric services alone cannot be the only ones to deal with mental health. The more psychiatric services work in an integrated manner with other agencies, formal and informal, the more effective the promotion of mental health will be. General Practitioners, public agencies, volunteers, families and patients associations, schools, etc. are some examples of other partners needed for the maintenance and promotion of mental health in the community. We described elsewhere the meaning of the de-institutionalisation process (Grispini, Piccione, 1998 b).

2. *The promotion of a new culture of mental health in school.* This means: a) to increase the awareness in the students regarding problems of mental health and reduce the stigma connected to psychiatric disorders and with psychiatric services, b) to enrich the relational opportunity and increase the ability of coping, c) to develop the teachers' skills to manage student-groups, d) to promote experiences of self-help, e) early identification of mental states at risk.

3. *The introduction of brief, economic and effective therapeutic tools to treat non severe mental disorders.* This means to stress, after a careful assessment of the patients and his *mileu*, the role of counseling, brief psychotherapies, large groups, self-help groups, all of these run alongside the more common technical measures.

4. *Early interventions in pre-psychotic phases and in mental states at risk* detected by the model of aggregation of risk factors in people who shows minimal but identifiable signs of distress (Mrazek, Haggerty, 1994; Yung et al.,1998).

References

Cozza M., Napolitano G.M. (1996) *L'assistenza psichiatrica in Italia: la normativa e la diffusione dei servizi sul territorio*, Istituto Italiano di Medicina Sociale Editore, Roma.

McGorry P. (1998) 'Verging on reality', *The British Journal of Psychiatry*, June, vol.172, Supplement 33.

Mrazek P.J., Haggerty R.J. (Eds), (1994) *Reducing risks for mental disorders*, National Academy Press, Washington, D.C.

Piccione R. (1994), *Proposte di psichiatria preventiva*, Bulzoni Editore, Roma.

Piccione R. et al. (1995) *Il processo di valutazione nel Dipartimento di Salute Mentale Roma E: anno 1995*, DSM ASL RME, Roma.

Piccione R., Grispini A. (Eds), (1998a) *Prevenzione e salute mentale*, Carocci Editore, Roma.

Piccione R., Grispini A. (1998b) 'Il modello preventivo: prospettive ed opportunità per lo sviluppo dei Dipartimenti di Salute Mentale', *Rivista Sperimentale di Freniatria* (in press).

Yung A.R., Phillips L.G., McGorry P.D., McFarlane C.A., Francey S., Harrigan S., Patton G.C. and Jackson H.J. (1998) 'Prediction of psychosis', *The British Journal of Psychiatry*, June 1998, vol.172, Supplement 33, 14-20.

12 'Mental Health': A Contested Concept

SANDY HERRON AND REBECCA MORTIMER

Abstract

The literature reflects a contested view of the concept mental health. What we 'know about' mental health can be translated within the definitions, models, elements of and criteria for mental health and within the language used to discuss 'mental health' itself. Although it is acknowledged these differing ways of knowing about mental health do not exist in isolation from one another they can offer a clear systematic and logical approach to reviewing the concept mental health. In doing this, however, it is clear that there is no common consensus as to what is meant by 'mental health'. Thus, the aim of this paper is to present an overview of these differing ways of knowing about mental health and to critically discuss the implications of having a contested concept.

Introduction

The literature reflects an understanding of mental health that is 'convoluted', 'ambiguous', 'controversial' and 'multi-faceted, personal and dynamic' in nature which it is argued, presents exactly the same problems in conceptualisation as 'health' (Eaton, 1951; Insel & Roth, 1979; MacDonald & O'Hara, 1996). In his early work Eaton (1951) argues that mental health is a 'conceptual abstraction' whilst Boorse (1976) contends that mental health is a 'web of obscurity'. In a similar vein, Sahakian (1970) points out that *'consensus regarding mental health is far from unanimous'*. Certainly Jahoda

(1958) has been cited on numerous occasions to have argued that:

> ...there is hardly a term in current psychological thought as vague, elusive and ambiguous as the term mental health (p.3).

Forty years on and researchers, theorists and practitioners a like still continue to contest the nature and meaning of mental health. The contested nature of mental health can be appreciated by examining the differing ways of 'knowing about' mental health itself. Writers have argued that the definitions, models, elements of and criteria for mental health and the way we use the language of mental health influences and offers insight into what and how we know about 'mental health' (Herron, 1998a). In essence, they provide 'windows' into the thoughts and beliefs (with respect to mental health) of the individuals who adopt them. These differing ways of knowing about mental health do not exist in isolation, they interact, inform and influence each other. However, in exploring these areas the convoluted, contested and largely ambiguous nature of mental health can be fully revealed.

Definitions of Mental Health

Definitions of mental health offer a conceptual snap-shot of how researchers, theorists and practitioners view mental health. Definitions encapsulate and reflect how differing cultures see mental health within specific temporal locations. For instance, Preston (1943) in an early definition defines mental health as:

> ...the ability to live happily...productively...without being a nuisance... (p.112).

More recent writers have argued more specifically that mental health is:

> ...(a) absence of dysfunction in psychological, emotional, behavioural and social sphere, (b) optimal functioning or well-being in these domains. (Kazdin, 1993).

Certainly, these two definitions reflect a common belief that mental health is usually thought of in terms of behaviours and experiences that conform to certain standards of functioning, rationality and even morality (Insel & Roth, 1979 p.55). However, their basic content and context may differ. For instance, some theorists and practitioners have adopted a life-cycle approach to defining mental health, its development and its promotion (for instance, Albee,

1994). Within this stance mental health is seen as being (a) *functional* (Kakar, 1984), (b) *relational* (Money, 1994), (c) to do with *ability* and *capacity* (Chwedorowicz, 1992) and (d) as *social* (Epp, 1988). Alternatively, mental health may also be viewed in terms of the principle of homeostasis (Menninger, 1963). Parkins (1994) further argues that mental health should be described in such a way that the mental qualities relate to the normal biological organisation of out species and so it should include physiologically based information concerning the normal development and functioning of the brain (p.288). Certainly, it is argued that definitions of mental health seldom meet with general approval (Dalzell-Ward, 1967). Although some may have similar features the term 'mental health' is difficult to specify. Some writers have argued that *'no universally accepted definition is available'* (Warr, 1987). A lay definition of mental health (see Herron, 1998a & b) supports the previously cited view of Shipman (1995) who argues that *'...mental health appears to be all things to all people...'* (p.4). Pulling together the all the threads to provide a static conceptual snap shot of how lay people view mental health is extremely difficult. As my own work reveals, the lay perspectives of mental health are not static, but dynamic and change in light of new experience, knowledge and social exchange. Moreover, there are a large number of main and sub-perspectives each reflecting a relativistic view of mental health. A lay definition of mental health would, in order to be holistic, need, for instance, to reflect notions of illness as well as wellness and notions of ability as well as inability. I argue that this alone leads to a contested definition of mental health and therefore ultimately ambiguities when it comes to mental health promotion.

Models of Mental Health

Models reflect an abstract representation of a reality/theory driven construct which act as analytic frameworks which can clarify thinking and guide practice. In essence, models are often designed (but not always) in an attempt to operationalise a definition of mental health. They can draw upon a number of definitions and are used to provide an 'image' of how mental health is to be viewed. However, it is this very point that provides the basis for a contested concept of mental health. Discrepancies between writers occur in the basic content of their definitions, the facts they address and the features they describe, as well as in terms of style (Warr, 1987). It is thus, rarely possible to integrate the definitions of mental health proposed by different writers. There are three main models of mental health within the literature. The first is the

105

unipolar model whereby mental health is merely seen as a euphemism for mental illness and thus, subsequently, also from within its derivative activities. Secondly, the *bipolar* model reflects a view that mental health is seen to exist on the opposing end of the same continuum as mental illness (Eaton, 1951). These two models, however, demand that mental health be, either directly, or by implication, viewed through a mental illness rather than a mental health lens - as a *secondary* concept (Trent, 1992). This in itself further deepens the contested nature of mental health. Although mental illness has been examined extensively from differing ontological and epistemological standpoints, it also remains again very much a contested concept (see Herron, 1998a pp 13-20). Thirdly, the two continua model contends that mental health is a separate and distinct concept to mental illness (MNHW, 1988). Despite its modern emergence, this model is based upon the early work of writers such as Jahoda (1958) who explored the positive nature of mental health and largely rejected the view that mental health was the absence of mental illness. She believed that mental health and mental illness are not correlative terms but separate entities and therefore should be treated as such. Within this model, mental health spans form minimal mental health to optimal mental health. As such it is considered to be the 'positive' mental health model due to its emphasis on the enhancement of human qualities for its own sake, rather than its value in disease prevention (MacDonald & O'Hara, 1996). Understanding mental health therefore demands a more salutogenic (health enhancing) rather than pathogenic (illness orientated) focus (Antonovsky, 1979). It is easy to see that within these three models alone lie contrasting viewpoints, which when translated into practice may create inconsistencies in both scope and intention of any mental health promotion strategy. Furthermore, within the two-continua perspective lie a number of sub-models, each reflecting possibly competing and contrasting views of mental health. Trent (1991) argues that mental health is a cable of inter-linking continua whereby the strands of illness and health are separate but closely related - hence reflecting a discrete yet interconnected nature of mental health. This model (although it is intended to show how external forces can influence an individual) tends to reflect an individualistic view of mental health. In contrast, the *map* model of mental health (MacDonald & O'Hara, 1996) reflects a much more social ecological perspective. I argue therefore, that the priorities given within each model further lend support to the argument that mental health is a contested concept. Since the lay perspectives of mental health are relativistic, any lay model of mental health must also reflect this. My own work identifies that a lay model of mental health reflects a holistic stance, in that it identifies the existence of both positive and negative images of mental health (see Herron, 1998 pp 255-256 and Herron, 1998c). Furthermore, it includes individual as well as social aspects of mental health. Therefore, within its very foundations a lay model of mental health would again reflect the contesting nature of mental health itself.

The Elements/Criteria of Mental Health

The elements of or criteria for mental health reflect the emphasis given to specific features of a definition or a model. Thus the presence of such elements inform the reader as to what characterises and/or 'constitutes' mental health. Here lies the point whereby the contested nature of mental health can be seen. The literature demonstrates that the elements of and/or criteria for mental health are complex. What is accepted as an indication of 'mental health' in one culture may not necessarily be accepted within another (Furnando, 1990). This reflecting the subjective and relativistic nature of mental health. It must be acknowledged that other writers have noted that the elements of or criteria for mental health should be treated as *descriptions* rather than *prescriptions* (MacDonald, 1992). However, what is understood by mental health is very much dependent upon which elements or criteria are given priority. For instance, happiness, it is argued by many (Argyle, 1987), is an indication of mental health. And whilst I can plausibly agree with this I do feel that since happiness is made up of so many other 'prime' factors, exactly what constitutes happiness (therefore, mental health) remains very much a matter of opinion. Trent (1991) in an attempt to isolate the basic content of mental health has looked towards identifying *enhancing elements* (such as accomplishment, challenge, competence, humour and trust) and *demoting elements* - namely, shame, guilt, fear and psychological isolation. Others have isolated elements that are more specific to an individuals ability to have a relationship with oneself, others and the environment (Money, 1994). However, again my own work on the lay perspectives of mental health has isolated elements such as spiritual intimacy; feelings of self-acceptance; a sense of belonging, the ability to work; the ability to be economically and socially productive; notions of control and empowerment; issues concerned with social support (emotional, practical and informational) and the ability to establish and maintain relationships (Herron, 1998a p.258). This is by no means an exhaustive list, the possibilities are endless. However, the pertinent issue here is that whilst these elements of or criteria for mental health aid our understanding as to what could be seen to be the 'building blocks' of mental health, they remain at times, competing and contesting.

The Language of Mental Health

The final way to 'know about' mental health, as reviewed within this paper, is to explore the interchangeable language used throughout the literature. When I was reviewing the concept mental health as part of my PhD work I found the language of mental health to be a minefield. Others have found similar patterns (Pavis et al, 1996). Terms such as subjective well-being, life satisfaction, happiness and quality of life have been used to indicate mental health. Writers such as Argyle & Martin (1991) and Hoyt and Creech (1983) have made attempts to draw tight definition boundaries around these concepts, whilst others have used the terms interchangeably with the term 'mental health' (Veenhoven, 1991). Similarly 'psychological', 'emotional' and 'spiritual health' are often used interchangeably with 'mental health' (see Tudor, 1996). Furthermore, the literature demonstrates that the term 'mental health' may be itself used as an integrative or generic term encompassing differing definitions of mental health. For instance, using Groder's (1977) octahedron model of mental health Tudor (1991:25) argues that mental health is an integrative concept covering terms such as 'emotional literacy', 'affective well-being', the 'emotional dimension of well-being', 'affective education', 'cognitive literacy' and 'somatic education'. As we have already seen, mental health is more commonly used interchangeably with terms such as 'mental illness' and specifically within the workplace as 'stress'. Notions of happiness and contentment have been expressed within lay studies (Pavis et al, 1996). Others identified that words such as depression and schizophrenia are readily used (Rogers et al, 1996). Terms such as 'nutter', 'insane', 'going off your trolley', 'holistic health', 'emotional health', 'being in balance' and 'a state of equilibrium' are also indicated (Herron, 1998a p.258). The language of mental health carries with it both positive and negative connotations. For example the lay perspectives of mental health shows that when mental health is used as a euphemism for mental illness images of fear, violence and distrust are generated. As a social constructions researcher I would argue that through language we create our reality and hence, our view of mental health. We invent concepts, models and schemes to make sense of experience, Furthermore, we continually test and modify these constructions in light of new experience. As such what we know about and how we influence each other in what they know about mental health is very much a product of social exchange. Therefore, isolating the language of mental health is very difficult, and I again argue may indeed underpin the contesting nature of mental health.

The Reality of a Contested Concept

The reality of all this, therefore, is that whilst significant progress towards actively promoting mental health has been achieved over the years, it can be argued that the main barrier to the development of effective and sustainable mental health promotion strategies and initiatives has been, and continues to be, the contested nature of the concept 'mental health'. Some writers have argued for the need to have a shared concept of mental health (Braidwood, 1996) whilst others have maintained that defining mental health is a fruitless exercise resulting in time spent arguing over semantics (Money, 1997). However, is it just a case of semantics or is there a need for a shared concept? I would probably have to agree with the latter. However, by this I do not argue for developing that ultimate definition or model of mental health. Nor do I adhere to the view that all the elements of or criteria for mental health could ever be isolated. And certainly I do not contend that the language of mental health could ever remain rigid enough to reflect a fixed view of mental health. I believe that just as with 'health' mental health **will** remain contested. There will never be a commonly held consensus from which **all** theorists, researchers and practitioners adhere to. It is like reducing all the people in the world into one single entity. However, I believe based upon this review, my current joint work with Dennis Trent and my own work within the lay perspectives of mental health that it is time to move towards accepting the contested nature of mental health. To see the contested nature of mental health as a quality and an opportunity rather than a problem. The very fact that mental health is contested provides us with a holistic framework itself from which to hang any strategy. However, the problem is that we need to pull together a framework which will incorporate the contrasting and competing views of mental health. As a result, create a framework from which we can as researchers, theorists and practitioners work side by side - not always within the same perspective, but with a sense that there are alternative ways in which things can be done. We need to put behind us the constant debates of what is mental health and move towards how can we operationalise a concept of mental health that incorporates and gives value to **all** the perspectives.

The Way Forward

I acknowledge that this needs a great deal of development and certainly an area in which I am currently working. However, I would argue that the way forward is fourfold. Firstly we need to acknowledge that mental health does, and will, continue to mean all things to all people. Secondly, I feel there is a need to accept this. Thirdly, to devise some framework that incorporates these differing ways of knowing about mental health. To accept that whilst some believe mental health is directly linked to mental illness, others argue for the closely inter-linked yet separate nature between mental health and mental illness. Fourthly, to isolate the prime factors common to these perspectives and to utilise them in constructing a form of tool which will monitor progress made in (a) strategies designed to reduce mental illness and (b) strategies designed to actively promote mental health (either within a bipolar or two continua perspective). I would argue that unless we create some flexible tool that can be applied within a holistic view of mental health we will never be able to evaluate the success of mental health promotion strategies. Indication of success will remain an 'illness' issue. Thus, we will never be able to lobby effectively for funding and priority for pro-active mental health promotion initiatives. This in its bare form may seem in itself a contesting issue – especially since I have argued for a tool that can be used both within an illness and a health framework. Certainly discussion of this is beyond the scope of this paper. However, this belief is derived from a view that rather than objecting to the contesting nature of mental health we should accept that alternative ways of looking at the world will always exist. Mental health, as with the concept health, has been, and will remain, subjectively based and hence, a contesting concept.

References

Albee, G. W. (1994) 'The fourth revolution', in Trent, D.R. and Reed, C. (eds.) *Promotion of Mental Health* (3) pp. 1-16 Avebury, Aldershot.

Antonovsky, A. (1979) *Health, Stress and Coping: New Perspectives on Mental and Physical Well-being*. Jossey-Bass, San Francisco.

Argyle, M. (1987) *The Psychology of Happiness*. Methuen, London.

Argyle, M. and Martin, A. (1991) 'The psychological causes of happiness', In Strack, F., Argyle, M. and Schwarz, N. (eds.) *Subjective well-being: An inter-disciplinary approach*. Pergamon, New York.

Boorse, C. (1976) What a theory of mental health should be. *Journal of the Theory of Social Behaviour*, 6(1): pp.61-84.

Braidwood, E. (1996) *In Search of a Shared Concept: An Exploration of the Concept of Mental Health Promotion*. Unpublished MSc Dissertation. Leeds University.

Chiu, H. (1992) 'Mental health and dualism', in Trent, D.R. (ed.) *Promoting Mental Health* (1):31 Avebury, Aldershot.

Chwedorowicz, A. (1992) 'Psychic hygiene in mental health promotion', in Trent, D.R. (ed.) *Promoting Mental Health* (1): pp. 24-26. Aldershot, Avebury.

Dalzell-Ward, A.J. (1967) 'Health Education for mental health', *Health Education Journal.* (26): pp. 192-203.

Eaton, J.W. (1951) 'The assessment of mental health', *The American Journal of Psychiatry.* (108): pp. 81-90.

Epp, J. (1988) 'Promoting the mental health of children and youth: Foundations for the future', *Canadian Journal of Public Health* 79(2): pp. 56-59.

Furnando, S. (1990) (Ed.) *Mental Health in a Multi-ethnic society: A Multi-Disciplinary Handbook,* Routledge, London.

Herron, S. (1998a) *Lay Perspectives of Mental Health.* Unpublished Ph.D. Thesis. Liverpool John Moores University, Centre for Health.

Herron, S. (1998b) *Defining Mental Health: The Lay Perspective.* (forthcoming) School of Nursing, Postgraduate Division, Faculty of Medicine, QMC, Nottingham University.

Herron, S. (1998c) *Towards a Lay Model of Mental Health.* (forthcoming) School of Nursing, Postgraduate Division, Faculty of Medicine, QMC, Nottingham University.

Hoyt, D. and Creech, C. (1983) 'The life satisfaction index: A methodological and theoretical critique', *Journal of Gerontology* (38): pp. 111-116.

Insel, P.U. and Roth, W. T. (1979) *Health in a Changing Society.* Mayfield Publishing Co.

Jahoda, M. (1958) *Current Concepts of Positive Mental Health,* Basic Books, New York.

Kakar, S. (1984) *Shamans, Mystics and Doctors: A Psychological Enquiry into India and its Healing Traditions,* Unwin, London.

Kazdin, A.E. (1993) 'Adolescent mental health: Promotion and treatment programs', *American Psychologist* 48(2): p. 127.

MacDonald, G. (1992) 'Defining the goals and raising the issues', in Trent, D.R. and Reed, C. (eds.) *Promotion of Mental Health* (2) Averbury, Aldershot.

MacDonald, G. and O'Hara, K. (1996) *Ten Elements of Mental Health in Promotion and Demotion: Implications for Practice.* Paper presented at the European Conference on the Promotion of Mental Health. London.

Menninger, K. (1963) *The Vital Balance: The Life Process in Mental Health and Illness.* Viking press, New York.

Minister of National Health and Welfare (1988) *Mental Health for Canadians.* Ottawa.

Money, M. (1994) 'Following the Shamanic pathway to mental health' in Trent, D.R. and Reed, C. (eds.) *Promoting Mental Health* (3) Avebury, Aldershot.

Money, M. (1997) Defining mental health: What do we think we are doing? *Positive Mental Health and its Promotion.* Liverpool John Moores University, Centre for Health. ISBN: 1 900248 15 8. pp. 13-15.

Parkins, E.J. (1994) 'Equilibrium and cognitive neuropsychology: Is mental health just a question of balance?' in Trent, D.R. and Reed, C. (eds.) *Promoting Mental Health* (3): pp. 287-303, Avebury, Aldershot.

Pavis, S., Masters, H. and Cunningham-Burely, S. (1996) *Lay Concepts of Positive Mental Health and How it Can be Maintained.* Final Report. Edinburgh, Department of Public Health Science, University of Edinburgh.

Preston, G.H. (1943) *The Substance of Mental Health*, Rinehart and Co. Inc., New York.

Rogers, A., Pilgrim, D. And Latham, M. (1996) *Understanding and Promoting Mental Health.* HEA, Family Health Research Reports.

Sahakian, W.S. (1970) (ed.) *Psychopathology Today.* Peacock Publishers.

Shipman, C. (1995) *Mental Health Promotion: A Review of Evaluations and Activities.* North Buckinghamshire Health Promotion Unit.

Trent, D.R. (1991) Breaking the single continuum. In Trent, D.R. (Ed.) *Promotion of Mental Health* (1) Avebury, Aldershot.

Trent, D.R. (1992) 'The promotion of mental health: Fallacies of current thinking', in Trent, D.R. and Reed, C. (1992) *Promotion of Mental Health* (2) Avebury, Aldershot.

Tudor, K. (1996) *Mental Health Promotion: Paradigms and Practice*, Routledge, London.

Veenhoven, R. (1991) 'Question of happiness: Classical topics, modern answers, blind spot', in Strack, F., Argyle, M. and Schwarz, N. (eds.) *Subjective well-being: An inter-disciplinary approach.* Pergamon, New York.

Warr, P. (1987) 'A Study of Psychological Well-being', *British Journal of Psychology* (69): pp. 11-121.

13 Lay Perspectives of Mental Health: A Summary of the Findings

DR. SANDY HERRON

Abstract

The aim of this paper is to give a broad overview of the findings of a recent three year Q method study designed to explore and explicate the lay perspectives of mental health. In order to contextualise the findings, this paper will begin by offering a very brief review of the concept mental health with specific reference made to the lay perspective. An in-depth look at the methodology has been documented elsewhere (Herron, 1998a & b) therefore, it is not the purpose of this paper to replicate this information. Henceforth only a brief summary of the background of the study and the steps taken will be offered. The seven lay perspectives of mental health found in the current study are summarised individually. This paper will then culminate with a critical discussion of the specific and wider implications of these findings both in relation to the existing knowledge of the lay perspectives of mental health and for mental health promotion in general.

Introduction

The lay perspectives of mental health have seldom been explored (except Pavis et al, 1996; Rogers, et al, 1996). Both these studies offer excellent insights into a relatively uncharted territory and are extremely useful in illuminating the lay view of the effects of relationships (either personal, intimate or professional) on mental health. These studies tended, however, to conclude that lay people find it difficult to think of and discuss mental health beyond the 'taken for granted'. Where explanation is given, mental health is located within the body, specifically within the brain. Furthermore, there is a tendency of individuals to adhere to the euphemistic (unipolar) (Pilgrim & Rogers, 1993) or the bipolar view of mental health (Eaton, 1951). Pavis et al (1996) argues that lay people have very little (if any) salience for the concept 'positive mental health' (the two continua model). Terminology used to discuss mental health tend to reflect notions of happiness and contentment. In contrast terms such as depression and schizophrenia are also readily used within lay discourse (Rogers, et al, 1996). In the main the findings reflect the existing belief that the lay perspectives of mental health are self evident and merely reflect those of the psychiatric hegemony (Waxler, 1977). Some writers have argued that where lay accounting differs from that of the professional, it is discredited as being unimportant or 'uniformed' and hence seen to be 'wrong' (Furnham, 1984). It has been argued that this has led to the lack of exploration of the lay perspectives of mental health (Herron, 1998a). However, this seems a little remarkable in the light of the enormous contribution that lay perspective studies have made to our understanding of health, illness (see Stainton Rogers, 1991) and mental illness (Gleeson, 1991). Research into lay health belief has established some degree of consensus that sophisticated lay models of explanation, distinct from biomedical ones do exist. Therefore, given this, and to bridge a gap in a new area, the initial aim of the research outlined here, was to explore the *lay perspectives of mental health*.

The Study

The study was conducted within the city of Liverpool between 1993 and 1996 (see Herron, 1998a & b). Two sample groups were targeted - namely, sample group one **(current mental health service users)** and sample group two **(current non-mental health service users)**. Much of the 'specifics' of the research were the direct result of research saturation within the city at the commencement of the study and also in response to local needs, targets and priorities. The age range was limited to the 18-30 age group. This was dictated by many of the services willing and available to take part. Both men and women were encouraged to take part. The study focused on the non-statutory sector only, again, a response to the existing mental health research climate within the city of Liverpool. A Q methodological approach was used. This was to combine to strengths of both quantitative and qualitative research traditions (see Herron, 1998c). To ensure the lay perspectives of mental health were explored within the day to day reality of the people of Liverpool, Q method avoided the imposition of a priori typical of quantitative research methods and the imposition of a posteriori typified by the qualitative methods (see Herron, 1998a pp. 59-60). This enabled the researcher to ask lay people what they thought mental health was without adhering to any pre-existing world view of mental health. Unstructured interviews were used to gather the initial data in stage one of Q method. Interview themes were devised by combining the findings from the pilot study with the findings from an extensive literature review. They were not asked verbatim, but rather used as triggers, to guide the interview. A total of 150 interviews were carried out. This represented a combination of one to one interviews and focus groups. Triangulation of the methods was encouraged by asking some participants to take part in both approaches. Analysis of the interview data was carried out by using a simple transferral technique (Brown, 1980) combined with a step by step process of analysis as outlined by Burnard (1991). This resulted in a list of 90 themes which reflected the broad content of the original interview material. Before the themes could be used within the Q set they needed to be reduced to statements by eliminating duplicates and merging similar themes. This was carried out using a consensually evolving approach to Q set construction (see Brown, 1980) followed by a process to ensure constructual validation by other researchers. The list of statements were piloted to ensure they adequately reflected the original interview data. Participants were asked to compare the list of statements against their original interview transcript. On completion and following modifications in light of the findings from the pilot study, a list of 58 statements was produced to form the Q set. This was then sent to all the participants for sorting according to salience. There was a response rate of 67% from both sample groups. The responses were analysed using PCQ3 (Stricklin, 1996) (each sample group was analysed separately owing to the constraints of the analysis tool). The 'product' of Q method was a total of **seven** factors which reflected seven perspectives of mental health.

The Findings

(1) The 'Illness' Perspective

This perspective was identified by **both** sample groups. It reflects a belief that mental health is merely seen as a euphemism for mental illness (the unipolar model). Mental health is therefore discussed in terms of early classi-

115

fication, intervention and treatment regimes. Within this mental health is seen to be more associated with women than men and therefore seen as an unwanted commodity. Lay people argue that within this perspective there are varying degrees of mental health, spanning from depression to schizophrenia. Mental health is expressed in negative terminology e.g. 'nutter', 'insane', 'bonkers', 'wacky'. This perspective is 'problem' orientated and expressed as 'inability to do...' or 'a lack of....'. It acknowledges the illness focus of the existing mental health services and argues for the need for services to look more at ways of *getting rid* of mental health. Mental health is not seen to be the responsibility of the individual - it is seen to be something that the services need to address. It is argued, perspectives of mental health are created mainly as a result of personal experiences and to a lesser extent by the media, family and friends and society at large. Least salience is given towards formal education.

(2) The 'Health' Perspective

Mental health is seen as a separate concept to mental illness. It is viewed as a wanted commodity and discussed in terms of 'being in balance', 'a state of equilibrium' and 'holistic health'. The process of becoming or being mentally health is given a much more salutogenic focus and is expressed by phrases such as 're-balancing', 'increasing personal awareness' and 'personal enlightenment'. In contrast to the 'illness' perspective, here mental health is seen as an 'ability to do...' (e.g. work) and/or 'having a sense of...' (e.g. self-acceptance). There also seems some common agreement that lay perspectives of mental health are created by the media (although identified that not always positive images are created), society at large and formal education. Least salience is given to personal experiences. This perspective was identified by **both** sample groups. However, whilst a common salutogenic thread runs between them the detailed perspective differs according to sample group.

Participants in **sample group two (non-service users)** argue that mental health, even though seen to have a different meaning to mental illness is, in fact, an opposing but related concept - a bipolar concept. Mental health is seen to exist on the opposite end of the same continuum to mental illness. Mental health is gained by moving along the continuum towards mental health and away from the mental illness end. Movement is the result of enhancing the positive elements of mental health and demoting elements of mental illness. A good supportive relationship is given identified as an enhancing element. In contrast, an unstable volatile relationship is given as a demoting element. Within this bipolar view of mental health, mental health is seen to

116

be more associated with women than men. It is argued that the rationale behind this is that women are more likely to attend mental health services, therefore, they have greater potential for moving towards the mental health end of the continuum. In a related vein, it is argued that changing the term mental health to 'emotional health' would not only result in an increased 'health' orientated focus of mental health services but would also encourage male attendance at these services. Participants argue further that mental health services have a tendency to be 'reactive' in nature - i.e. only there for when things go wrong. However, there seems to be an acceptance that this is necessary and appropriate, whilst arguing for the need for mental health service providers to look for more ways to also actively promote mental health.

In contrast, participants in **sample group one (service users)** argue that within the health perspective of mental health lies a view that mental health is a completely separate and distinct concept to mental illness (the two continua model). Varying degrees of mental health are seen to exist within this perspective. They range from minimal mental health to optimal mental health. There is a non-dependency relationship between mental health and mental illness. Neither concept depends upon the existence or absence of the other for its own existence. Furthermore, it is argued that both men and women have equal potential for mental health. The reactive nature of existing mental health services is strongly acknowledged. It is argued that in order to promote mental health there is definitely a need for services to re-focus and hence develop health enhancing strategies.

(3) The 'Purchaser-Provider' Perspective

Identified by **both** sample groups. Lay people see a dichotomy between the individual *(purchaser)* and the service *(provider)* perspective of mental health. It is argued that lay people see mental health as a separate concept to mental illness (two continua). In contrast, service providers are seen to view mental health within a unipolar perspective. Furthermore, service providers are seen to adhere to the illness view of mental health. Services are problem orientated in cognitive, behavioural and physiological dimensions. They are reactive and curative in focus. Lay people argue that this leads to a 'gap' in service provision between what is needed and wanted and what is actually delivered. This lay perspective of mental health argues for a need to view mental health as a separate concept to mental illness, to re-focus services so that promotion is given equal priority to prevention - with the ultimate goal to be 'pro-active' in promoting mental health.

117

(4) The 'Public-Private' Perspective

This perspective was identified by **both** sample groups. Here mental health is seen within both a 'health' and an 'illness' perspective. However, this perspective argues that there is a public - private divide in accounting for mental health. It is argued that individuals are afraid to voice their 'true' perspective when the dominant and prevailing perspective is an illness one. This, infers that people may frequently view mental health from a health framework but are unwilling to disclose their view in public. Fear seems to be related to fear of being ostracised or being seen as 'different'. We have seen a public-private difference in accounting within the research interview situation, however, this perspective takes it out of the interview arena and puts it within the wider social content and context.

(5) The 'Exemption' Perspective

Offered by participants of sample group one (service users) only. In a similar light to the purchaser - provider view of mental health, this perspective offers a dichotomous view of mental health. The dichotomy stems from the acknowledgement of both the 'health' and the 'illness' perspectives. There is also an acknowledgement that mental health can be viewed both as a wanted and unwanted commodity. It is this very dichotomy which provides the foundations for this perspective. When mental health is seen as a euphemism for mental illness and all its derivative connotations it is argued that the term itself is used to legitimise certain role exemptions such as work. Mental health is not interchanged with the term mental illness here, but more accurately, with the term stress. It is argued that due to the increasing acceptance that stress is a product of our urban pace of life, and hence not the responsibility of the individual, then stress no-longer carries with it stigma or taboo as would have been reflected in previous years. Therefore, in this way, mental health is in some cases very much a wanted commodity for its legitimised exemption properties.

(6) The 'Relationship' Perspective

Identified by participants in sample group two (non-service users) only. Initially it appears to be paradoxical in that both the health (bipolar in this case) and the illness perspectives of mental health are rejected. Participants argue that this is because neither perspective is 'right' or 'wrong' since it is dependant upon the perspective held. This perspective argues for a link between the identified perspective of mental health and relationships. As with other lay perspective work of this kind there is a clear view that the term relationship may encompass an intimate sexual relationship with a partner of any gender or it may be a close relationship with a friend or family member. However, it is argued that being able to establish and maintain a relationship (despite its nature) could indeed, within the lay perspective, be a 'marker' of mental health. Certainly, being seen to be mentally healthy is seen to be a pre-requisite for a relationship. Otherwise, there is fear of being 'tarred with the same brush', which it is argued is not conducive for a solid lasting relationship. This also reflects the belief when mental health is viewed in terms of mental illness there are unfavourable connotations associated with it. The actual effects of a relationship on mental health is also discussed. Relationships may act as a 'buffer' militating against the development of mental illness. Alternatively, relationships may act as an enhancer for the maintenance and/or development of positive mental health. In contrast, relationships may also act as an enhancer for mental illness, especially when the relationship is volatile, unstable and uncaring.

(7) The 'Religion' Perspective

As with the relationship perspective his perspective initially appears to be paradoxical. However, unlike the former, both the health (bipolar in this case) and illness perspectives are accepted. This perspective argues for a link between religion and mental health. When mental health is seen as a euphemism for mental illness, religion is seen to act as a buffer militating against the development of the same. In contrast when mental health is seen as a bipolar concept to mental illness there is a commonly held view that religion is seen to promote mental health. The buffering and promoting nature of religion stems from people having a greater sense of belonging and acceptance. Through religious activity religion may (a) provide greater social contact, (b) reduce social isolation, (c) offer potential for greater social support (actual and perceived), (d) increase the possibility of finding a confidant, (e) increase feelings of solidarity and cohesiveness, (f) strengthen friendship and family and (g) offers individuals a purpose in life - which it is argued, provides the *essence* of positive mental health. This perspective recognises the usual interchange between 'religion' and 'spirituality'. However, the buffering and promoting effects of the latter provides spiritual intimacy through prayer. Prayer itself provides a means for coping. It is argued people who pray have an increased sense of security (feelings of being protected by God).

Implications for the Existing Lay Perspectives

The findings demonstrate that the lay perspectives of mental health are convoluted and at times contradictory. They are wide and ranging and address
issues concerned with the (a) the lay view of the concept mental health itself,
(b) the factors which promote, demote or maintain 'mental health', (c) offers
glimpses of the use of language of mental health within lay discourse, (d)
informs the gender-mental health debate, (e) the influence of relationships on
mental health and vice-versa, (f) the link between mental health and religion,
(g) it offers insights into the lay view of current mental health services and
(h) provides a lay view of the required future direction of service provision.
However, the main implication of the findings is that they contest some of the
previously held views of the lay perspectives of mental health. It is argued
that lay people are able to think and discuss mental health beyond the taken
for granted. Their perspectives, although at times complex, demonstrate that
indeed lay explanations of mental health do exist and can inform the overall
debate. Certainly, the findings confirm the three main models of mental health
reflected within the professional arena. However, what is of more importance
here, is the salience towards the concept 'positive mental health'. It is argued
that since participants were allowed to identify their own perspective of mental health, this then facilitated isolating an understanding of mental health
that parallels the view reflected within the two continua model (c.f. Pavis et
al, 1996). This contests a previously held assumption within the existing knowledge of the lay perspectives of mental health. Furthermore, little (if any) reference was made towards mental health being located within the body. Individual content was implied, however, these findings placed mental health
also within the social content and context. As such, views of mental health do
seem to be actively constructed and negotiated in light of new experience,
knowledge and through the daily process of social exchange. Henceforth, the
lay perspectives of mental health are not merely watered down versions of
professional discourse but reflect the construction of individually and col-
lectively informed models of explanation. Whilst there is an acknowledgement that the professional may indeed inform the lay view, the findings contend that the process is not a passive one, rather it is dynamic and relativistic.
As such it is argued that lay perspectives of mental health are not 'self-evi-

dent' but rather they offer surprising and fruitful insights into the concept mental health.

Implications for Mental Health Promotion

Whilst it is acknowledged that work on the lay perspectives of mental health is in its infancy the lay voice may offer some direction for mental health promotion. The findings clearly identify that promotion of mental health ought to receive equal attention (and funding) to mental illness prevention. Mental health service providers need to re-dress the focus. There is a need to develop strategies that focus upon mental health from within a two continua as well as bipolar perspective. Re-education of professionals may be necessary. World mental health days may need to focus upon promoting a positive view of mental health rather than solely focusing upon for instance, defeat depression campaigns. Whilst these are important they also reflect an 'illness' view of mental health. To conclude, whilst mental health has been extensively addressed over the years (albeit from differing epistemological and ontological standpoints) there is a need to explore further the lay perspectives of 'mental health'. As the findings infer, there is a need to accept the relativistic nature of mental health and to move towards isolating ways of combining the lay and the professional view so that, not only, can mental illness be prevented, but also mental health be actively promoted.

References

Brown, S.R. (1980) *Political subjectivity: Applications of Q method in political science.* Yale University Press, New Haven & London.

Burnard, P. (1991) 'A method of analysing interview transcripts in qualitative research', *Nurse Education Today* (11): pp.461-466.

Eaton, J.W. (1951) 'The assessment of mental health', *The American Journal of Psychiatry.* (108): pp. 81-90.

Furnham, A. (1984) 'The lay conceptions of neuroticism', *Personal and Individual Differences.* 5(1): pp. 95-103.

Gleeson, K. (1991) *Out of our minds: The deconstruction and reconstruction of madness.* Unpublished P.D. Thesis. University of Reading.

Herron, S. (1998a) *Lay perspectives of mental health. Unpublished Ph.D.* Thesis. Liverpool John Moores University. Centre for Health.

Herron, S (1998b) Lay perspectives of mental health: A Q method study. Submitted to *The Sociology of Health and Illness.*

Herron, S. (1998c) Researching mental health: Q versus ethnography. *Submitted to Journal of Health Psychology.*

Pavis, S., Masters, H. and Cunningham-Burley, S. (1996) *Lay concepts of positive mental health and how it can be maintained.* Final Report. Edinburgh. Department of Public Health Science. University of Edinburgh.

Pilgrim, D. and Rogers, A. (1993) *A Sociology of Mental Health and Illness*, Open University Press, Buckingham.

Rogers, A., Pilgrim, D. and Latham, M. (1996) *Understanding and Promoting Mental Health*, HEA, London.

Stainton Rogers, W. (1991) *Explaining Health and Illness*, Wheatsheaf, London.

Stricklin, M. (1996) *PCQ3 (Version 3b).* Computer Software. USA.

Waxler, N.E. (1977) 'Is mental health cured in traditional society? A theoretical analysis', *Culture, Medicine and Psychology* (1): pp. 233-255.

14 Men and their Travails: Breaking the Silence

KEN KEDDIE

In the past men, by virtue of the work they did, as farmers, miners, soldiers and the like, were able to experience lives filled with purpose and comradeship. The arrival of new technology over the past few decades has caused a social revolution marked, for example, by high levels of unemployment and early retirement. The women's movement has focused people's minds on many of the traditional ideas about gender. A few decades ago women began to question their role as traditional care-takers for the family. A practical consequence of the change in thinking has been the increased, and still rising, number of women in employment. Men will have to alter their thinking and their behaviour in order to survive these changes, as the sense of identity and of integrity that came from being in work is no longer guaranteed.

Until my recent retirement I worked as a psychiatrist and in that setting I was aware that society had had to date relatively little interest in men's welfare. In my clinical practice I was witness on many occasions to the demolition of men's self-esteem. Current health statistics confirm these impressions of mine. They demonstrate that men's health compares poorly in many respects with that of women:

- Men die, on average, 5 years before women
- Men are 4 times more likely to commit suicide
- The young male suicide rate has increased by 75% in the last 10 years
- Men under 65 are 3.5 times at risk of coronary heart disease compared to women
- Men are twice as likely to die of lung cancer

- Men are responsible for 90% of violence with 66% of victims being other men
- 88% of court appearances are made by young men
- 66% of intravenous drug-users are male
- Alcohol misuse is predominantly male
- Sexually transmitted infections (including HP!) occur mostly in men
- Gay men are routinely discriminated against socially and legally.

All this demonstrates that men are suffering and dying, unnecessarily and prematurely, in large numbers. Indeed these casualties can be likened to the fallen on some massive, wearisome battlefield: a pitiful and protracted latter-day Verdun unfolding behind a facade of normality. Men also suffer disproportionately when partnerships or marriages are dissolved in terms of access to their children. In such circumstances 50% of fathers lose contact with their offspring after two years.

For some time I have felt that a medical approach to psychological malaise in men is, on its own, inadequate. For this reason I began to pursue an interest in a community approach to men's issues, including those of alcohol and drug related problems. Violence is another well known pursuit of men. Indeed many men have a finely tuned facility for humiliating and dominating. The following passage from the Universal Declaration of Human Rights, promulgated exactly 50 years ago, reminds us how far we still have to progress in this regard:

> No-one shall be subjected to torture or to cruel, inhuman or degrading treatment or punishment.

Aggression in men has, of course numerous causes, but one of the most significant of these may be the feeling of resentment that emanates from parental betrayal through lack of love, attention and guidance. The father-son relationship is often flawed, perhaps because the type of closeness that existed formerly, the older man and the younger man working together side by side in the field and the workshop, no longer obtains.

Men need to work hard in order to redress the demonizing of the father. Reconciliation is eventually possible and the solution is in our own hands. Indeed the American poet Wallace Stevens reminds us of "the son who bears upon his back/The father that he loves, and bears him from/The ruins of the past, out of nothing left."

Men have a deep reservoir of pain and anger. They find intolerable the inherited model of masculinity, which trains men to repress their emotions and to focus instead on external success. There is a perpetual process of con-

124

ditioning to act in a barbaric manner which men undergo as they grow up.

In order to survive the ordeal of having been wounded, in a psychological sense, many men adopt a confrontational pose. Other men try to defend themselves by becoming critical, or demeaning, towards others. Some simply try to protect themselves by withdrawing into newspapers, television, booze or work.

Men these days yearn to be validated, not for their traditional roles of providing, protecting and procreating, but as human beings able to embrace a new kind of manhood, which allows them to be nurturing and reflective. They would then be able to see themselves as people able to listen, relax, rejoice, enthuse. They would be able to enjoy each other's company and each other's conversation. It is through such personal contact and free-flowing dialogue that we learn to be comfortable with ourselves. We thereby discover who we are and also the particular meaning that life has for us. This credo stresses the vulnerability of men, as well as their strengths, and opposes the intimidation of women, children and other men.

But pious hopes about improving men's well-being are not enough. There is a conspiracy of silence about the difficulties that face men today. The outcast status of contemporary man has been left off the political agenda altogether. Well ... almost left off ... for now we are beginning to hear encouraging words from our politicians on men's issues.

Paul Boating, MP, Parliamentary Under-Secretary for Health, urged us yesterday at this conference to recognize that men have a need at times to talk on a meaning level with other men. This is sadly a need that is so often unmet. When such mutual support is available, it helps, in my opinion, to bolster men's sense of well-being and to enhance their mental health.

Also, in to-day's newspapers it is reported that Jack Straw, the UK Home Secretary (The Times, 1998) has spoken of the Government's plans to set up a national family and parenting institute, Straw suggests that men should be encouraged for one thing to get together in "Dad's Groups" in order to discuss the emotional and practical problems of raising children . He views favourably the idea of "mentoring" projects, where older men - i.e. men with stable family lives - would provide one to one support for troubled youngsters with no father figures in their background.

The Government is also looking at ways of providing practical help for grandparents supporting families.

To correct the frequent apathy then, let us look at other practical initiatives, at local and national levels. For men themselves have to assume responsibility for their lives. There is no alternative. Men need to explore fresh ways of helping themselves. They have to become more aware of the malign influence of, what I call, the masculine siege mentality. This phenomenon is characterised by isolation, an uneasiness in the world of emotion, a prefer-ence for action over discourse, addictive behaviour, an opting for confronta-tion rather than collaboration, an approach that regards creativity as effete and a bewilderment at society's a la mode views on gender relations.

Feminism, with the force and energy of its radical political outlook, has compelled both men and women to question whether or not the ideal family is one that is economically independent, socially responsible, law-abiding and observant of contemporary norms (Grayling 1997). Faced with this high-profile public debate, many men find themselves mesmerized and disheart-ened.

I believe that networking amongst men, at a personal as well as an infor-mation-technology level, presents a challenging and realistic way of healing the current emotional blight that affects men. This could come about more easily by the formation of local MEN'S CIRCLES OF FRIENDSHIP. Such gatherings would provide a supportive ambiance in which to share mutual concerns and to explore relevant issues. From my experience, I find that such milieu.x afford men the opportunity to explore, along with others, the wis-dom that emanates from literature and poetry. This can often lead to insights that are helpful and inspiring.

Men's Circles of Friendship would encourage men to discover, or re-discover, their worth through their own efforts. One consequence might be the emergence of what Blaise Pascal (Pascal 1965) calls "hommes honnetes", i.e. measured and attentive men of all round excellence, who impose neither boastfulness nor arrogance on others.

To celebrate the creation of such Circles of Friendship, a suitable logo

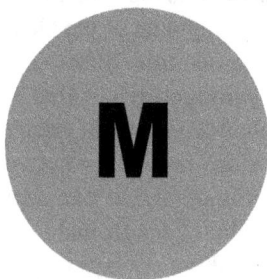

might be devised, perhaps in the form of a forest-green letter M on a cerulean blue background.

(dark green M on a light blue background)

126

These colours, Nature's own, are echoes of everlasting images of foliage framed against cloudless skies.

In his book, "The Future of Men" (Will 1997), will emphasises the positive aspects of manhood: adventurousness, physical courage, risk-taking, rugged individualism. Will contrasts these attributes with the sorry state of affairs, whereby the growing youth has to learn the rules of manly conduct "He will be expected to taunt or be taunted, bully or be bullied, destroy or be destroyed. He will be expected to conform to the codes of the male group or be ruthlessly excluded from it". Will concludes his treatise perceptively with these words: "There is a sense in which the future of men was started by women. Now men must do some of the work. They should begin at the beginning: with themselves and with their sons.

I vigourously applaud these sentiments and, furthermore, I would like to a think that the changes in perception and attitude, that males must adopt in order to survive and flourish, will slowly gather momentum as the years unfold.

Mulling over such considerations, I recently penned the following poem for the youngest of my three grandsons to mark his first birthday:

Anthology for a Grandson

be bold young man
be bold
throughout your life
be bold

let not the tyrants ways
distort
dismay
unfettered be and free

be firm young man
be firm
make time to understand
to weigh the pros and cons
before you speak your mind
and envy not
the sharpened tongue
and waspish wit

what's real

127

is not your neighbour's view
but yours
and yours alone

be still young man
be still
make time
to stop and stare
to view the ever-changing scene

the drifting clouds
that paint an artist's dream
the jets of rain
that freshen field
and path alike
and there
triumphant in the sky
an arc
of endless hues

be true young man
be true
hold friendship dear
lose not the gentle touch
the understanding smile

affirm each day
your deep humanity
a light you'll be
in other people's lives

and to yourself be true
indulge at times
in waywardness
abandon not the zest of youth
press on and dance with glee

be bold young man

be bold

              be firm
                be still
                    be true

but

most of all

be you

Of all the arts, poetry, in particular, enables us to ask ourselves fundamental questions concerning the great permanent themes of love, nature, loss,
death, religion: What are we doing here? How can we deal with fear and pain
and sorrow? Where can we find comfort? While poetry offers no certain answers, it can "console us and sustain us" (Matthew Arnold) and bring us "a
clarification of life" (Robert Frost) (Antis 1973). Poetry is as necessary a part
of ourselves as it was for past civilisations. Robert Graves got to the heart of
the matter by describing poetry as "heartrending sense".

Poetry allows us not to feel alone as we tackle the evils of cruelty and
injustice. Once we stop considering, and re-considering, what constitutes the
world around us, there is a real danger of slipping into mindless barbarism.

The poet's ear responds to the rhythmic flow of words and his or her soul
vibrates to the whispering breeze, the babbling brook, the swaying trees, the
smiling child, the loving heart of a friend and the inward voices that speak of
the life beyond.

Such inspiration is all around us. Recently I chanced on "A Subaltern's
Musings", a book of poems written by Hamish Mann (Mann 1915). Man was
an officer, who served in the Black Watch, and who was seriously wounded
on 9th April 1917 whilst leading his platoon in the advance at Arras, North
France. He died the following day, barely 21 years of age. Mann's poems,
written mostly in the trenches, were published posthumously in 1918. His
verses remind us that it is the life that is simple and uncomplicated that is
worth living:

This is what *I* ask: the sky above;
  The wind's caress;
The joys of Friends; or, when I need it,
  Loneliness.

In January 1914, in Edinburgh, some eighteen months before he was
gazetted, he wrote the poem, "Friendship", perhaps mindful of the comrade-

ship that would sustain him in the conflict to come.

Friendship

There are few things more beautiful than Friendship
    good and true;
There are few names more beautiful than "Friend",
In Friendship there are mingled Love, Respect, and
    Pleasure too, -
In it the laws of true Religion blend.

I have my Friend: - I can defy the Earth!
    Hence, dull and carking Care, and foolish Love!
There is no joy in this wide world that's worth
    The gift of Friendship, sent us from Above.

We owe it to Hamish Mann and his like to order our lives somewhat differently. A fellow poet and kindred spirit, Kahil Gibran cautions us with these words:

... let there be no purpose in friendship save the deepening of the spirit
(Gibran 1976).

In this way men will achieve accommodation with other men by looking beyond the distractions and trumperies of everyday life. Once more let Blaise Pascal be our guide. To my mind, he hints at the direction to be followed in his Pensees "L' homme n'est qu'un roseau":

Man is only a reed, the weakest in nature, but he is a thinking reed. There is no need for the whole universe to take up arms to crush him: a vapour, a drop of water is enough to kill him. But even if the universe were to crush him, man would still be nobler than his slayers, because he knows that he is dying and the advantage the universe has over him. The universe knows none of this. Thus all our dignity consists in thought It is on thought that we much depend for our recovery, not on space and time, which we could never fill. Let us then strive to think well; that is the basis of morality.

I wish now to turn to my second suggestion with respect to combating contemporary man's isolation. One difficulty is that there is no effective organisation to forge appropriate remedies. For this reason I am keen to promote the idea of REGIONAL MEN'S FORUMS, comprising farseeing, sunpatico men and women from all walks of life. These forums would serve the purpose of collating information relating to men's mental health, of influencing public opinion and of encouraging the enactment in parliament of appropriate legislation.

At a practical level, Regional Men's Forums would have to make recommendations about the type of support needed for those men, who are vulnerable, in order to reduce their sense of alienation and worthlessness. Participants would have to be alive, of course, to the activist, political dimensions that characterise today's men's movements in the U.K. For many people, men and women, believe that feminism has strayed too far from the original, worthy pursuit of achieving equality with men, but that it now indulges in the cultural vilification of men.

The day will come when both authoritarian masculinity and militant feminism are outmoded forces in society. At that point people will be permitted to be their authentic selves. In order for that to be realised men and women have to be encouraged to participate together in a constructive and civil type of gender politics. It is in this way that a world, noted for its tolerance of diversity and fairness for all human beings, will eventually be created.

References

Amis, Kingsley (1973) 'Why Poetry?' *Observer Magazine* 30 Sept. 1973 p. 39.
Gibran, Kahil (1976), The Prophet, p. 70, Heinemann, London.
Grayling, A. C. (1997) *The Future of Moral Values,* p.17, Phoenix, London.
Mann, Hamish (1918) *A Subaltern's Musings*, John Lang, London.
Pascal, Blaise. 1965. *Pensees*, Larousse, Paris.
The Times (1998), Straw Proposes 'fathers' unions', 10 Sept. 1998, p.2.
Will, Dave (1997) *The Future of Men,* pp. 54-55, Phoenix, London.

Acknowledgements

In the compilation of this paper I wish to acknowledge support from:

Michael Easton

Jake Hensman

Trevor Johns

Ann Keddie

Ian Keddie

James Kennedy

Margaret Kennedy

Jim Kiddie

Billy McCall

Pam McDougal

Millar Mair

Norman Piercy

Alastair Reid

James Scott

Paul Scott

Suzanne Sheridan

David West

15 The Need for Supportive Strategies for the Person who Self-Harms

KATHRYN KINMOND

Abstract

The stated target reduction in annual suicide-rates was 15% by the year 2000, (*Health of the Nation* White Paper 1992). It was noted that this could be achieved if the number of people completing suicide within a year of presenting to A&E with Deliberate Self-Harm (DSH), were to be halved (Royal College of Psychiatrists 1994). The latest government White Paper (*Our Healthier Nation*, 1998) sets a target reduction in annual suicide-rates of one-sixth by 2010. The close links between suicide and DSH (Williams & Morgan 1994), emphasise the importance of effective psychosocial assessment for all people presenting to A&E with DSH. Yet fifteen years after the DHSS circular (LASSL(84)5), first criticised the high levels of discharge without psychosocial assessment, of people presenting to A&E with DSH, concerns are still being raised. To assist hospitals, The Royal College of Psychiatrists published a consensus statement on standards of service for the general hospital management of adult DSH (CR32 1994), but to date, there is no definitive approach to service provision. This paper reviews the literature and details two West Midland hospitals, which currently adopt different approaches to the care of the individual who deliberately self-harms. The paper concludes by reviewing some of the problems and questions which remain unanswered, in this highly emotive area.

Introduction

The target reduction in annual suicide-rates of 15% by the year 2000 (*Health of the Nation (1992)*, Department of Health), could be achieved if the number of patients completing suicide within a year of presenting to A&E with DSH, were to be halved (Royal College of Psychiatrists 1994). The close links between suicide and DSH (Kreitman & Foster, 1991: Williams & Morgan 1994), emphasise the importance of effective psychosocial assessment for all people presenting to A&E with DSH.

In the UK estimates of the prevalence of deliberate self harm (DSH), vary between 0.4% and more than 10% of the general population (Favazza and Rosenthal, 1993; Babiker and Arnold, 1997). Whichever estimate is closer to reality, DSH is common and its frequency makes it a major public health concern. In 1984, the Department of Health and Social Security (DHSS), stated that DSH accounted for the highest acute medical admissions for women and the second highest for young men (LASSL(84)5). No further statistics on medical admissions for DSH, have been published, by what is now the Department of Health; however, ten years after the original paper by the DHSS, Hawton estimated that over 100,000 people present to Accident and Emergency departments (A&E), for DSH in England and Wales every year (Hawton, Fagg, Simkin & Mills 1994). The recent shift towards care in the community for people with a diagnosed mental illness means that hidden within these data are also psychiatric patients, presenting with DSH to A&E, perhaps during a crisis. Though this group is not identified specifically within the overall DSH statistics, Draucker (1992) notes that many patients attending A&E with diagnosed mental illness, are those who repeatedly harm themselves.

In 1984, the DHSS (LASSL(84)5), suggested that patients who harm themselves should be assessed and followed up by a multi-disciplinary team. Their recommendations considered for the first time, the employment of professional workers other than psychiatrists to follow-up referrals from 'suitably trained practitioners'. This document followed closely that of the Standard Nursing and Midwifery Committee (SAC(N) (84) 22), which suggested in a letter to the Royal College of Psychiatrists, that Community Psychiatric Nurses have an important contribution to make to the after-care of this group, in conjunction with other workers in the community. Yet almost fifteen years later, the DHSS's recommendations are still to be effected as policy. Sidley and Renton (1996), emphasised the responsibility of each NHS Trust to put in place a multi-disciplinary team, in order to meet the needs of both the health-care staff and the individuals presenting with DSH. Further, Greenwood and Bradley (1997), suggested that the way forward is to involve a multi-disciplinary team, consisting of doctors, nurses, psychiatric and other services to investigate protocols to deal with assessment, referral and possible discharge of patients. In 1984, the DHSS (LASSL(84)5), criticised hospital services that discharged patients before they had been assessed psychosocially. Yet in 1995, Hawton commented that the frequent discharge of patients following DSH episodes from A&E departments, without a basic psychosocial assessment, should be a cause for great concern. Arguably, service provision for those presenting with DSH to A&E, has progressed little in fifteen years.

Greenwood and Bradley (1997) note variance in discharge rates between patients presenting with physical DSH (categorised as self-inflicted wounds) and those presenting with poisoning. Their audit of one hospital, showed that of those harming themselves physically, 40% were discharged home, with only 25% being referred to acute psychiatry. Of those self-poisoning, 16% were discharged home, with 70% admitted to hospital for psychiatric assessment. Kapur (1998) suggested that bed shortages mean that DSH patients are often not likely to be admitted because they are deemed neither to be at great physical risk nor suffering from severe mental illness, which would necessitate admission to a psychiatric bed. This 'low-risk' is often determined by A&E staff, without psychosocial assessment of the patient.

Concerns over effective psychosocial assessment of individuals presenting to A&E following DSH, led The Royal College of Psychiatrists to publish a consensus statement on standards of service for the general hospital management of adult DSH (CR32 1994). This document noted that *despite the scale of DSH, planning and delivery of services are in disarray locally and nationally* (p4), with no definitive approach to service provision. The document laid out 'ideal standards' against which providers might measure their service, taking as a premise, the fact that assessment and management of DSH patients might be undertaken by staff other than psychiatrists. Following publication of this document, some Trusts have undertaken their own clinical audit of both numbers of individuals presenting with DSH and also the service provided.

Audits of Two West Midland Hospitals

Data collected by two acute hospitals in the West Midlands, provided a very similar picture of patterns of DSH presentations to A&E, but the two hospitals have responded in very different ways to the care of these individuals.

Both hospitals operate an A&E department into where most individuals presenting with DSH as an acute medical admission, are taken. If patients are referred by a General practitioner, they attend the Medical Admissions Unit, though this accounts for only 5% – 10% of cases.

In their audits, both hospitals recorded approximately 2 attendances for DSH to A&E, per day. By far the most common method recorded, was overdosing, with over 85% of cases for each hospital. Physical harm was recorded for approximately 10% cases. There was a relatively even sex-distribution recorded for both hospitals with the majority of attendances (over 75%), for individuals aged between 15 and 65 years. Discharge-rates were also similar for both hospitals:

Hospital A:

- 19% were repeating DSH.
- 46% were admitted into hospital.
- 54% were discharged home; the decision having been made by staff on A&E.

Hospital B:

- 5% were repeating DSH.
- 52% were admitted into hospital, with 37% being referred for formal psychosocial assessment.
- 43% were discharged home; this decision having been made by staff on A&E.
- 5% were transferred from A&E to other hospitals; their needs being assessed as requiring care not offered by the Hospital.

These audits enable only limited cross-tabulation of data and further work is currently being carried out at both hospitals.

Following the audit and other work, each hospital has adopted a different approach to the care and management of the patient presenting with DSH. Hospital A implemented a liaison psychiatry service, commencing in December 1996; hospital B, decided against this provision initially, preferring to purchase psychiatric services. However, a proposal for a community psychiatric nurse specialist (CPN), based within the Home Treatment Team, to be on-call for patients presenting with DSH to A&E, is currently being reviewed. The proposed system will depend on initial screening and referral by

A&E staff, with the designated CPN then carrying out formal psychosocial assessment. Additionally, access to the Home Treatment Team should facilitate effective utilisation of resources and ensure that other suitably qualified and experienced CPNs are available to liase with A&E staff and DSH patients as required.

There are clearly documented difficulties associated with caring for the person presenting with DSH (Patel 1975; Ghodse 1987) particularly within the culture of A&E (Duffy 1993; McLaughlin, 1994). Liaison psychiatry is a recent response which promotes the interface between general psychiatry and medicine and a number of Trusts now operate this system, though the team and its remit are structured in various ways. Evans, Cox and Turnbull (1992) documented their model, initially set up at King's Cross Hospital in 1986. Common to most liaison psychiatry services, is initial screening and referral by A&E staff, with liaison psychiatry, usually a multi-disciplinary team, then carrying out formal psychosocial assessment. The liaison psychiatry service at hospital A comprises of one Consultant Liaison Psychiatrist, one Senior House Officer (SHO), one Liaison Nurse Manager, four nurses with RMN training and a secretary. Until recently there was also an occupational therapist. Social work support is accessed through Mental Health Services. The liaison psychiatry service, for patients aged 16 and over, operates on a daily basis between 9.00 a.m. and 10.00 p.m. Outside these times, the on-call doctor is contacted and referral to liaison psychiatry is made as appropriate, the following day. Individuals under the age of 16, are referred to Child and Family Services.

Work currently being undertaken will evaluate both hospitals' approaches to service provision.

The 'Survivors' Movement

Outside the medical response to caring for the individual who self-harms, the last ten to fifteen years has seen a growth in the 'user' or 'survivors' movement, through organisations such as the Bristol Crisis Centre for Women, the Basement Project and the National Self-harm Network. The Bristol Crisis Centre for Women was initially set up in 1986 to support women in emotional distress, but from the outset, it was clear that DSH was an area in which support and understanding were particularly needed. The organisation developed a focus in DSH and began promoting better public and professional understanding of the issue. The Basement Project, also based in Bristol, provides training, consultation and publications in DSH for individuals and those working in community and mental health services. The National Self-Harm Network is a survivor-led organisation, founded in 1994, committed to campaigning for the rights and understanding of those who self-harm. All these organisations offer support and understanding different from that provided by the medical services. Additionally, they are influencing care within medical services by opening dialogue and giving suggestions for protocol; for example, nursing individuals presenting with DSH, is increasingly through triage. Nursing and medical staff in A&E are frequently the health practitioners who have most involvement with individuals in the period immediately following a self-harm episode and their attitude towards, and treatment of, the individual, is important. It has also been noted as being influential in terms of future episodes of DSH (Arnold 1995).

Articles about DSH are increasingly to be found in the psychiatric, psychological and independent literature. The Henderson Hospital hosted two conferences in 1997, attended by over 800 delegates, many from various sectors of the health service. The scale of the interest in DSH is clear. There has also been exploration within the media; though as Fiona Lynn (1998) reports, this is not always helpful. For example, Channel 5 chose to portray DSH as having strong links with tattooing, body-piercing and food-disorders (June 1998: *Damage)*. Yet despite the scale of the interest, the whole debate surrounding DSH remains confused and contentious. The varied use of terminology and difficulties with clarifying associated attributions further complicate an already complex area and a definition of DSH, acceptable to both 'professionals' and 'survivors', remains elusive. This lack of consensus has implications both for constructive discourse and also for sharing of best practice and many questions remain unanswered.

Some Questions Remaining

For example, who presents to A&E and what about those self-harming who do not seek medical attention? Favazza and Conterio (1989); Babiker and Arnold (1997), note that DSH is underreported. In their community survey, Favazza and Conterio found that 39% of individuals self-harming, said that they had not sought medical treatment for their injuries/poisoning. The reasons for this may only be guessed, but possibly the guilt and shame surrounding what is essentially a little- understood form of behaviour might dissuade a person from seeking medical help – particularly if the injury is not life-threatening. Additionally, a percentage of individuals will seek medical treatment, either at hospital or via their G.P, with injuries/poisoning described as 'accidental', which in reality will have been DSH (Arnold and Magill 1998).

All these individuals will remain 'hidden' from any official statistic and hence, those documented 'officially', may represent only a limited sample of the total numbers of individuals involved.

Some individuals perceive DSH as a personal coping strategy in times of extreme distress, emphasising the importance of the *functions* of and *motivation* behind some forms of DSH. Rather than viewing the DSH as destructive, this perspective suggests that DSH *can be said in some ways to be carrying out the very reverse of self-destructiveness...rather than wishing to destroy themselves, their self-injury helps them to stay 'together', to struggle to survive* (Babiker & Arnold, 1997 (p7)).

Arnold's (1995) survey of women who self-harm, also supports the view that DSH fulfils many important survival functions. In this context, intervention is unwanted and irrelevant, unless the harm becomes medically dangerous. Further, if individuals do not want to stop the behaviour, the health-care practitioner has neither the legal or moral justification to impose treatment. However, if they do not seek to intervene, what should the role of the health-care practitioner be?

And what about the realities of caring for individuals presenting with DSH to A&E?

The National Self-Harm Network (1998), reports that A&E staff may feel anger and frustration when the same person returns, having repeated the DSH and helpless, because no matter what they do, the harming continues. Additionally, many junior staff are at the 'cutting-edge', possibly before they have acquired life experience to support their medical skills and training. McLaughlin (1994), explored variable influencing attitudes of nursing staff in A&E. He found some correlation between the nurse's age and/or length of service and attitude towards DSH; with more understanding and empathy shown by experienced nurses. Duffy (1993) suggests that lack of appropriate training may inhibit effective care and supporting this, recent articles in the Nursing Times have documented the need for training in the care and support of individuals who self-harm, particularly for staff in A&E. By far the most commonly reported issue for women in their contact with medical services, was the attitude of staff. Arnold (1995), stated that women repeatedly told of being *criticised, ignored, told-off, dismissed as attention-seeking, a nuisance or wasting time (p18),* and individuals often 'do the rounds' so they're not remembered. Effective treatment from their perspective suggested overwhelmingly that, *A more accepting, non-judgemental response,* is the key to effective and sensitive care. Arnold (1995; p.27). Threatening withdrawal of treatment or applying the 'no-self-harming' contract advocated as a standard intervention in the USA (Egan 1997), is at best unsupported empirically and at worst, very destructive.

Conclusion

The frequency of DSH makes it a major public health concern, with estimates of over 100,000 presentations to Accident and Emergency departments (A&E), in England and Wales every year (Hawton, Fagg, Simkin and Mills 1994). Yet there is no definitive approach to service provision for this group nationally. The links between DSH and suicide are well-documented, (Williams & Morgan 1994), and emphasise the importance of effective psychosocial assessment for all people presenting to A&E with DSH. Yet the discharge rates for these individuals are still high and a matter of concern, (Hawton 1995). DSH is a complex, confused and often confusing form of behaviour and there are as many questions remaining as those for which we have answers. Interest in the area is growing and dialogue between the 'professionals' and 'survivors', offers the hope of a more *subjectivist, holistic, bottom-up and user-informed position* (Frost 1995), for service provision. However, further evaluative work needs to be undertaken to review service improvements; not simply in the context of prevention of suicide and repetition of DSH, but also from the perspective of the service-users and their understanding and experience of health-care. In this way a fully-informed and integrated approach might be adopted and implemented effectively, to the satisfaction of both users and providers.

References

Arnold, L. (1995) *Women and Self injury*. Bristol Crisis Centre for Women, Bristol.

Arnold , L and Magill, A. (1996) *Working with self-injury*. The Basement Project, Bristol.

Arnold, L. and Magill, A.(1998) *What's the Harm?* The Basement Project, Bristol.

Babiker, G. Arnold, L. (1997) *The language of self-injury*. BPS Books.

Department of Health and Social Security (1984) Management of deliberate self-harm. *LA. SSL(84)5* London: HMSO.

Department of Health (1992*) Health of the Nation.* HMSO, London.

Draucker, C.B. (1992) *Counselling survivors of childhood sexual abuse.* Sage, London.

Duffy, A. (1993) 'Preventing suicide', *Nursing Times 89, p. 31.*

Egan, M., Riviera, S., Robillard, R., Hanson, A. (1997) 'The 'no-self-harming contract': helpful or harmful?', *Journal of Psychosocial Nursing; 35: 3, pp.31-33.*

Favazza, A.R. (1987) *Bodies under Siege: Self-mutilation in Culture and Psychiatry,* John Hopkins University Press, Baltimore, MD.

Favazza, A.R. and Conterio, K. (1989) 'Female Habitual Self-Mutilators', *Acta*

Psychiatrica Scandinavia, 79, pp.283-289.

Favazza, A.R. (1989) 'Why Patients Mutilate themselves', *Hospital and Community Psychiatry*, 40.2. pp. 137-145.

Frost, M.J.(1995) *Self-Harm and the social work relationship*, Social Work Monographs, Norwich.

Ghodse, A.E. (1988) 'The attitudes of casualty staff and ambulance personnel towards patients who take drug-overdoses', *Social Science and Medicine 12 pp.341-346.*

Greenwood, S. Bradley, P. (1997) 'Managing deliberate self harm: the A and E Perspective', *Accident and Emergency Nursing (1997) 5, pp. 134-136.*

Hawton, K. and Catalan, J. (1987) *Attempted suicide*, Oxford Medical Publications: Oxford.

Hawton, K. and Fagg, J. (1988) 'Suicide and other causes of death following attempted suicide*', British Journal of Psychiatry, 152: pp. 359-366.*

Hawton, K., Fagg, J. Simkin, S. and Mills, J. (1994) 'The Epidemiology of attempted suicide in the Oxford area, England (1989 - 1992)', *Crisis 15(3): pp. 123-135.*

Kapur, N. House, A. Creed, F. et al (1998) 'Management of deliberate self-poisoning in adults in four teaching hospitals: descriptive study', *British medical Journal; 316: 7134, pp. 831-832.*

Kreitman, N. (1977) *Parasuicide*, Wiley, Chichester.

Lynn, F. (1998) 'The pain of rejection', *Nursing Times 94, p. 27.*

McLaughlin, C. (1994) 'Casualty nurses' attitudes to attempted suicide', *Journal of Advanced Nursing*, 20 : pp. 1111-1118.

National Self-Harm Network (1998) *Advice for AandE Staff,* National Self- Harm Network, London.

Patel, A. (1975) 'Attitudes towards self-poisoning', *British Journal of Advanced Nursing*, 20. pp. 1111-1118.

Peterson, L.G. and Bonger, B. (1990) 'Repetitive suicidal crises: characteristics of repeating and non-repeating suicidal visitors to a psychiatric emergency service', *Psychopathology,* 23 (3) pp. 136-45.

Platt, S. (1992) 'Epidemiology of suicide and parasuicide', *Journal of Psychopharmacology* 6, pp. 291-299.

Royal College of Psychiatrists, London (1994) *The General Hospital Management of Adult Deliberate Self-Harm.* C32.

Sidley, G. Renton, J. (1996) 'General Nurses' attitudes to patients who self-harm', *Nursing Standard*, 10, 30, pp. 32-36.

Standard Nursing and Midwifery Committee (1984) *Guidance on the Management of Deliberate Self-Harm*, SAC(N)(84)22 DHSS 1984.

Williams, R. and Morgan, H.G. (1994) *Suicide prevention: the challenge confronted. A Manual of guidance for the purchasers and providers of mental health care*, HMSO, London.

141

16 Implementing Mental Health Promotion: A Health Education and Promotion Perspective

GERJO KOK

Abstract

Mental health promotion may learn from the achievements in the field of health education and promotion. Health education and promotion has seen four major developments in the last decades: the need for planning, the need for evaluation, the behaviour-environment issue, and the use of theory. A recently presented protocol for developing theory-based and evidence-based interventions, *Intervention Mapping,* is described here in more detail. Prominent in planning models and intervention protocols is *implementation.* The same expertise and professionalism that we put in the development of health promotion interventions for our target groups should be put in implementation interventions for program users and decision makers.

Introduction

The fields of mental health promotion and health education and promotion have been developed separately for a long time. Only recently some exchanges are made. Health education and promotion has learned from mental health theories such as relapse prevention theory (Marlatt and Gordon, 1986), the transtheoretical model of stages of change (Prochaska, et al., 1997), and theories on coping and self-management (Lazarus, 1993). Mental health promotion may in turn profit from some of the achievements in health education research and practice. In this paper we will present some perspectives from health education and promotion that could be useful for mental health promotion. We will specifically focus on the implementation phase, which is a relevant topic in health education. However, unfortunately, relatively few empirical studies are available (Oldenburg et al., 1997).

Planned Health Education and Promotion

Health education and health promotion are means to reach goals, one of which is prevention. Health education is specifically based on learning experiences in relation to behaviour change, health promotion is more generally related to changes in behaviour and the environment (Green and Kreuter, 1991). The field of health education and promotion has seen four major developments in the last decades: the need for planning, the need for evaluation, the behaviour - environment issue, and the use of theory.

The Need for Planning

To define clear goals and select adequate means, we need planning. Green and Kreuter (1991) suggest a series of planning steps: analysing the problem, analysing the behavioural and environmental conditions, analysing the determinants of those conditions, developing the intervention, and implementing the intervention. Then the steps are proceeded in the reverse order for evaluation. An example (Schaalma et al., 1996a): Aids/HIV infection is a serious problem. One of the relevant behavioural conditions is condom use by adolescents. The major determinant for consistently using or not using condoms is self-efficacy related to negotiating with the partner about condom use. The appropriate intervention is self-efficacy improvement by skills training and the appropriate implementation of this intervention takes place in schools by teachers. It may also be clear from these analyses, that school programs which focus on knowledge improvement will not have much effect.

In the planning model, certain behaviours may be represented by categories of behaviour, such as coping, self-regulation, or decision making. In general, self-regulatory behaviours can be categorised as: monitoring, evaluation, and action (Lazarus, 1993). Environmental conditions may be represented by role agents behaviour (see the environment-behaviour discussion later). The analysis of determinants of individual behaviour will be supported by social-psychological knowledge; the determinants of role agent's behaviour will additionally be supported by knowledge from organisational and political

144

sciences. In the example, the focus is on individual behaviour. However, in other countries, the availability and accessibility of condoms may be a serious barrier for consistent condom use. In that case the focus should be on environmental changes: making condoms cheaper and easier accessible. Finally, implementation is an essential element of planning and often underestimated. We will return to that issue later.

Planning is crucial in health promotion: the top failure in intervention development is to jump directly from the problem recognition to an intervention without completing the necessary steps in between, such as finding relevant psycho-social determinants other than health reasons (e.g. lack of skills in stead of lack of health knowledge).

The Need for Evaluation

The second major development in health education that followed the focus on planning, was the focus on evaluation (Rossi and Freeman, 1993). Clear goals and means lead to clear criteria for effect and process evaluation. Which also means that evaluation is not the end of the planning process but is an integrated part of planning from the start. A planned health education and promotion intervention should aspire to be more effective than a condition with the standard intervention, not just better than a control condition where there is no intervention. A badly planned intervention does not even deserve to be evaluated (Rossi and Freeman, 1993, p. 218). Process evaluation provides target persons' and implementers' evaluations. Effect evaluation provides comparisons between the intervention condition and a base-line or control condition.

Schaalma et al. (1996b) report that their carefully planned HIV prevention intervention was more effective than the standard HIV prevention activities, with respect to all determinants, especially self-efficacy, and with respect to reported risk behaviour. Students liked the program, as did teachers. That last fact is relevant for future implementation, as we will see later.

Anticipating evaluation is essential for health promotion: on the one hand the intervention objectives should be completely clear (e.g., 'students are confident that they can negotiate condom use with their steady partner'), but on the other hand the objectives should be feasible within the time frame of the evaluation study (e.g. increase in self-efficacy in stead of reduction in HI V-infections).

145

Health education has traditionally developed interventions for individual change. Over time, the influences of environmental factors became clearer. Some problems are directly caused by environmental conditions, such as air pollution, while many behaviours are primarily caused by external determinants, such as availability of condoms or product safety. The behaviour-environment discussion has a long history in health education and promotion (see McLeroy et al., 1988 versus Green et al., 1994). Bartholomew et al. (1998) suggest a practical solution: the environment is extremely relevant, but changes in the environment may be seen as decisions by agents, or as role behaviour, at various levels. Next to the individual level, there are the interpersonal, organisational, community and societal level, each having their own agents, such as health care professionals, managers, City Council, or politicians. For instance, Flynn et al. (1998) analysed politicians' intentions, attitudes and normative beliefs relative to voting on youth tobacco prevention legislation and suggested specific interventions at the societal level. There is some confusion in the health education and promotion literature on the relation between environmental conditions for the problem and external determinants of the behaviour. Bartholomew et al. (1998) state that this distinction is irrelevant as long as the intervention is directed at the environmental or external decision-makers.

Many problems need multi-level interventions, not only health education in the traditional sense. For instance, drunken driving can be reduced by frequent alcohol controls, the availability of alternative possibilities for traffic, and by carefully planned health education interventions, that focus on personal risk perception and on self-efficacy improvement for resistance to social pressure. Another example of an intervention directed at the environment is needle exchange program for the prevention of HIV with Injecting Drug Users. At the individual behaviour level, we try to get drug users to participate. Before that, we have to convince political decision makers (societal level) that needle exchange programs are actually preventing HIV and not promoting drug use (Vlahov and Junge, 1998). That environmental level change may be much more difficult to achieve than the individual behaviour change of drug users. We also have more empirical data on determinants of drug users' decisions than on politicians' decisions. Many health promoters have translated the recognition of environmental influences in a so called ecological approach in their interventions, often by community development and participatory methods (Minkler and Wallerstein, 1997).

Theories are a very important tool for professionals in health education and promotion. On the one hand, theories have become available to health promotion practice through textbooks such as Glanz et al. (1997). On the other hand, the application of theory has been a challenge for a long time, for researchers as well as practitioners. Students of health promotion learn of theories and learn how to apply theories to well selected practical problems. However, in real life the order is reversed: the problem is given and the practitioner has to find theories that may be helpful for better understanding or changing behaviour (Kok, et al. 1996). Recently, a protocol was published that describes a process for developing theory-based and evidence-based health education programs: *Intervention Mapping* (Bartholomew et al., 1998). As Intervention Mapping is a relatively new protocol that might be relevant for mental health promotion too, we will describe it in more detail below.

Intervention Mapping

Intervention Mapping distinguishes five steps: define proximal program objectives, select theoretical methods and practical strategies, design the program, anticipate adoption and implementation, and anticipate process and effect evaluation. Bartholomew and colleagues see planning as an iterative process: two steps forward and one step back.

Tools

Bartholomew et al. (1998) describe three core processes for Intervention Mapping, tools for the professional health promoter: searching the literature for empirical findings, accessing and using theory, and collecting and using new data. From the literature search, a provisional list of answers is developed, which is often not adequate in finding solutions for the problem. The planner must go further to search for theory, using three approaches: issue, concept and general theories approach. The *issue approach* searches the literature for theoretical perspectives on the issue. The *concept approach* begins with the concepts in the provisional answers, linking these concepts to theoretical constructs and theories that may be useful. The *general theory approach* considers general theories that may be applicable. Finally, it is important to identify

147

gaps in the information obtained and collect new data to fill these gaps.

Intervention Mapping Steps

The first step in Intervention Mapping is the development of proximal program objectives, a crossing of performance objectives, determinants and target groups. For instance, one proximal program objective for an HIV-prevention program in schools would be: "adolescents (target population) express their confidence (determinant) in successfully negotiating with the partner about condom use (performance objective)". Performance objectives are the specific behaviours that we want the target group (or the environmental agents) to 'do', as a result of the program. For example in the case of HIV prevention: buy condoms, have them with you, negotiate with the partner, use them correctly, and keep using them (Schaalma et al., 1996a; 1996b). Or in the case of coping with Cystic Fibrosis: watch, discover, think and act (Bartholomew et al., 1993). Determinants of behaviour can be personal or external. Personal determinants are, for instance: outcome expectations, social influences, and self-efficacy expectations. External determinants are, for instance: social norms and support, barriers. Target groups can be subgroups of the total group, for instance: men/women, people in different stages of change. Proximal program objectives are numerous and should be ordered by determinant. So we end this step with a series of lists, for instance, all proximal program objectives that have to do with skills training.

Intervention mapping step 2 is the selection of theoretical methods and practical strategies. The theoretical method is the technique derived from theory and research to realise the proximal program objective; the strategy is the practical application of that method. For instance the method for self-efficacy improvement could be modelling, the strategy could be peer modelling by video.

Intervention Mapping step 3 is the actual designing of the program, organising the strategies into a deliverable program and producing and pretesting the materials. In the example of HIV-prevention in schools, the program existed of five lessons, an interactive video, a brochure for students and a workbook for teachers (Schaalma et al., 1994).

A solid diffusion process is vital to ensure program success. So, in Intervention Mapping step 4 a plan is developed for systematic implementation of the program. The first thing to do, actually at the start of intervention development, is the development of a *linkage system,* linking program developers with program users. Then, an intervention is developed to promote adoption and implementation of the program by the intended program users. It may be clear that the anticipation of implementation is a relevant process from the very beginning of planning, not only at the end.

Finally, Intervention Mapping step 5 focuses on process and effect evaluation. Again, this process is relevant from the start, not only at the end. For instance "adolescents express their confidence in successfully negotiating with the partner about condom use" is an objective, but is also a measure of that objective, that can be asked in pre and post interviews with experimental and control group students.

Theories

We agree with McGuire's (1991) statement that "all theories are right". For a health education practitioner, the academic debate between defenders and opponents of a particular theory is not very relevant. What is relevant is the contribution of any theory to finding solutions for practical problems. Professional health educators will not limit themselves to only one or a few theories; practical problems may be approached from a multitude of theories, some of which the professional will discover for the first time. A number of theories have been shown to be useful in health education practice (see Glanz, et al., 1997; Connor and Norman, 1996). For the development of performance objectives: theories on Self Management and Coping (Lazarus, 1993), theories on Self-Efficacy (Bandura, 1997). For the analysis of determinants of behaviour and environmental conditions (or decision makers' behaviour): Theory of Planned Behaviour (TPB, see Montaño, et al., 1997; Connor and Sparks, 1996), Social Cognitive Theory (SCT, see Baranowski, et al., 1997; Schwarzer and Fuchs, 1996), the Trans-Theoretical Model of Stages of Change (TTM, Prochaska, et al., 1997). For the development of the intervention: Self Efficacy theories, SCT, TTM, Goal Setting theory (see Strecher et al., 1995), Relapse Prevention theory (Marlatt and Gordon, 1986), Community Development theory (Minkler and Wallerstein, 1997), Organisational Change theories (see Goodman, et al., 1997). Finally, for the anticipation of implementation: SCT, Diffusion of Innovations theory (see Oldenburg, et al., 1997). This list may be seen as a start for the general theories approach (see 'Tools'), however, that is the third and last of the theory-finding strategies. The professional health educator should first try to find theories through the issue- and concept-related approach, selecting theories that are not in this list or in the standard health promotion theories books. For instance, a search for theories on how to prevent discrimination of people with HI V/Aids will lead to specific theories on emotional reactions that cannot be found in the earlier mentioned references (see Dijker et al., 1997).

149

Implementation

Implementation is an essential element for any health promotion intervention. However, the issue of implementation is not studied adequately at this moment. We will distinguish between implementation by the program users and implementation by the decision maker.

Implementation by the Program User

An example is a teacher who is asked to use (implement) the AIDS-prevention program for schools. Orlandi (1986) introduced the so called *linkage group, a* group of program developers and program users, at least their representatives. It is important to have adequate representatives of the program users involved in the development of the intervention, from the start. They will be able to give feedback on plans and ideas, and they may develop a sense of ownership of the final product. An example: in the (Dutch) AIDS-prevention program, the developers wanted to include peer teaching as a result of the many reviews that supported the effectiveness of that method. However, the Dutch teachers were not familiar with peer teaching as an educational method and refused to introduce peer teaching for the first time in their class rooms with a sensitive topic as AIDS prevention. The linkage group wisely decided to leave out peer teaching. Had the developers included peer teaching, the program users would have cancelled that part, or even the whole program.

The implementation process is often depicted as a four step process (Rogers, 1983).

- dissemination: knowing that the program exists;
- adoption: having the program; implementation:
- using the program and
- institutionalisation: keep using the program.

In practice, the percentage of program users decreases with every step. The institutionalisation step is often only observed in a very small percentage of the potential program users (Paulussen et al, 1994). Program users have their own reasons for implementing or not implementing a program. Paulussen et al. (1995) studied the reasons for implementing AIDS-prevention programs by Dutch teachers.

Diffusion was positively related to participation in teacher networks.

Adoption was related to instrumentality of the program, especially if students would like the program. Implementation was related to the self-efficacy of the teacher about using the program in the classroom. Institutionalisation was related to school policy and involved the principal and the school board in stead of the teacher. Most surprisingly to the authors, the empirically shown effectiveness of the program was not influential at all, but expected students' reactions were. Interventions to promote implementation try to improve the progress through the implementation process. Unfortunately, the evidence about effective methods is lacking (see Parcel et al., 1989 for an exception). In the example of AIDS-prevention in schools, diffusion could be promoted by models that increase the visibility of the program. Adoption could be improved by models that increase expected outcomes of the program, especially students' approval. Implementation can be promoted by mutual adaptation of the program in the development process, using linkage. Institutionalisation may be improved by reinforcements and social support feedback.

Implementation by Decision Makers

An example is a local government deciding to continue (implement) an HIV prevention program for gay men through the local health service. Implementation decision makers may be a local government, a worksite management, or a sport association board. Health promoters do not always recognise that adopting an intervention by organisations means a change in that organisation (Goodman et al., 1997; Rogers, 1983). And to change an organisation, one needs to understand how an organisation works. Decision makers have their own goals and their own agendas. There are bureaucratic and political factors that compete with health promotion activities. Decision makers basically strive for stability, and often for power, both of which priorities are not necessarily related to health promotion priorities. We know that our target population is not rational in decisions about health, so it should not be a surprise that decision makers are not rational in their decisions about implementation of health promotion interventions. Policy development by decision makers is a small steps process, that often involves key people at various levels in the organisation, and where the participants try to avoid risks. Health promotion interventions should fit in with the relevant priorities in the organisation (Sabatier and Mazmanian, 1980). Many health promotion intervention developers lack political insight in the reasons that decision makers have for implementing or not implementing a health promotion intervention. The study by Flynn et al (1998) on legislators' voting behaviour, is a rare exception. Implementation at the decision making level can be promoted by

151

including the decision makers in the *linkage* group and by anticipating barriers for implementation. The same theoretical knowledge and empirical research protocols that we have available for changing our target groups' risk behaviour, can be applied to changing the decision makers' implementation behaviour.

Conclusion

Health education and promotion and mental health promotion can learn from each other. Health education and promotion has much to offer in terms of systematic planning, careful evaluation, recognition of environmental influences and the development of environmental interventions, the optimal application of theories and protocols for developing health promotion interventions using theories and evidence, such as: Intervention mapping. Prominent in planning models and intervention protocols is the anticipation of implementation: no intervention is going to be effective when it is not implemented on a large scale.

Implementation can be stimulated by implementation interventions. The same expertise and professionalism that we put in the development of health promotion interventions for our target group, should be put in implementation interventions for the program user and the program decision maker.

References

Bandura, A. (1997) *Self-efficacy:the exercise of control,* Freeman, New York.

Baranowski, T., Perxji, C. L. and Parcel, G. S. (1997) 'How individuals, environments, and health behaviors interact; social cognitive theory', in: K. Glanz, F.M. Lewis and B.K. Rimer (eds), *Health behavior and health education: Theory, research and practice, 2nd ed.* (pp. 153-178), Jossey Bass, San Francisco, CA.

Bartholomew, L. K., Sockrider, M. M., Seilheimer, D. K., Czyzewski, D. I., Parcel, G. S. and Spinelli, G.S. (1993) 'Performance objectives for the self management of Cystic Fibrosis', *Patient Education and Counseling* 22, pp. 15-25.

Bartholomew, L. K., Parcel. G. S. and Kok, G. (1998) Intervention Mapping: a process for designing theory- and evidence-based health education programs. *Health Education and Behavior,* 25, 545-563.

Connor, M. and Norman, P. (eds) (1996) *Predicting health behavior; research and practice with social cognitive model,*. Open University Press, Buckingham.

Connor, M. and Sparks, P., (1996) The theory of planned behavior and health behaviors.

In: M. Connor and P. Norman (eds), *Predicting health behavior; research and practice with social cognitive models* pp. 121-162, Open University Press, Buckingham.

Dijker, A. J., Koomen, W., and Kok, G. (1997) 'Interpersonal determinants of fear of people with AIDS: The moderating role of predictable behavior', *Basic and Applied Social Psychology,* 19, pp. 61-79.

Flynn, B. S., Goldstein, A. O., Solomon, L. J., Bauman, K. E., Gottlieb, N. H., Cohen, J. E., Munger, M. C., Dana, G. S. (1998) 'Predictors of state legislators' intentions to vote for cigarette tax increases', *Prevention Medicine,* 2, pp. 157-165.

Glanz, K., Lewis, F.M. and Rimer, B.K. (eds) (1997) *Health behavior and health education: Theory research and practice, 2nd ed,* Jossey Bass, San Francisco, CA.

Goodman, R. M., Steckler, A. and Kegler, M. C. (1997) 'Mobilizing organizations for health enhancement; theories of organizational change', in K. Glanz, F. M. Lewis and B. K. Rimer (eds), *Health Behavior and Health Education: Theory research and practice, 2nd ed.* (pp. 287-312) Jossey Bass, San Francisco, CA.

Green, L. W. and Kreuter, M. W. (1991) *Health promotion planning; an educational and environmental approach,* Mayfield, Mountain View, CA.

Green, L. W., Glanz, K., Hochbaum, M., Kok, G., Kreuter, M. W., Lewis, F. M., Long, K., Morisky, D., Rimer, B. K. and Rosenstock, I. M. (1994) 'Can we build on, or must we replace, the theories and models in health education?', *Health Education Research,* 9, 397-404.

Kok, G., Schaalma, H., De Vries, H., Parcel, G. and Paulussen, Th. (1996) 'Social psychology and health education', in: W. Stroebe and M. Hewstone (eds), *European review of social psychology, Volume* 7 (pp. 24 1-282), Wiley, Chicester, UK.

Lazarus, R. S., (1993) 'Coping theory and research: past, present, and future', *Psychosomatic Medicine,* 55, pp. 234-247.

Marlan, G. A. and Gordon, J. R. (eds) (1985) *Relapse Prevention,* Guilford Press, New York.

Mazmanian, D. A., Sabatier, P. A. (1980) *Effective policy implementation,* Lexington Books, Lexington.

McGuire, W. J. (1991) 'Using guiding-idea theories of the person to develop educational campaigns against drug abuse and other health threatening behavior', *Health Education Research,* 6, pp. 173-184.

McLeroy, K. R., Bibeau, D., Steckler, A., and Glanz, K. (1988) 'An ecological perspective on health promotion programs' *Health Education Quarterly* 8, pp. 351-377.

Minkler, M. and Wallerstein, N. (1997) 'Improving health through community organization and community building', in: K. Glanz, F. M. Lewis and B. K. Rimer (eds), *Health behavior and health education; theory research and practice, 2nd ed.* (pp. 241-269), Jossey-Bass, San Francisco, CA.

Montaño, D. E., Kasprzyk, D. and Taplin, S. H. (1997) 'The theory of reasoned action and the theory of planned behavior' in K. Glanz, F. M. Lewis and B. K. Rimer (eds), *Health behavior and health education: Theory research and practice, 2nd. ed.* (pp. 85-112), Jossey Bass, San Francisco, CA.

Oldenburg, B., Hardcastle, D. and Kok, G. (1997) 'Diffusion of health promotion and education programs', in K. Glanz, F. M. Lewis and B. K. Riner (eds.), *Health behavior and health education: Theory research and practice, 2nd ed.* (pp. 270-286), Jossey Bass, San Francisco, CA.

Orlandi, M. A., Landers, C., Weston, R. and Haley, N. (1990) 'Diffusion of health promotion innovations', in K. Glanz, F. M. Lewis and B. K. Rimer (eds), *Health behavior and health education: Theory research and practice* (pp. 288-313), Jossey Bass, San Francisco, CA.

Parcel, G. S. , Taylor, W. C., Brink, S. G., Gottlieb, N., Basen-Engquist, K., O'Hara-Tomkins, N., and Erikson, M. P. (1989) 'Translating theory into practice: Intervention strategies for the diffusion of a health promotion innovation', *Family and community Health,* 12: pp. 1-13.

Paulussen, Th., Kok, G. and Schaalma, H. (1994) 'Antecedents to adoption of classroom-based AIDS education in secondary schools', *Health Education Research,* 9, pp. 485-496.

Paulussen, Th. G. W., Kok, G., Schaalma, H. P. and Parcel, G. S. (1995) 'Diffusion of aids curricula among Dutch secondary school teachers' *Health Education Quarterly* 22, 227-243.

Prochaska, J. O., Redding, C. A. and Evers, K. E. (1997) 'The transtheoretical model and stages of change, in K. Glanz, F. M. Lewis and B. Rimer (eds), *Health behavior and health education; theory research and practice, 2nd ed.* (pp. 60-84), Jossey-Bass, San Francisco, CA.

Rogers, E. M., (1983) *Diffusion of innovations,* Free Press, New York.

Rossi, P. H. and Freeman, H. E. (1993) *Evaluation; a systematic approach, 5th edition,* Sage, Newbury Park, CA.

Schaalma, H., Kok, G. and Paulussen, T., (1996a) 'HIV behavioral interventions in young people in the Netherlands' *International Journal of STD and AIDS, 7 (suppl. 2),* pp. 43-46.

Schaalma, H., Kok, G., Bosker, R., Parcel, G., Peters, L., Poelman, J. and Reinders, J. (1996b) 'Planned development and evaluation of AIDS/STD education for secondary school students in the Netherlands: Short term effects', *Health Education Quarterly,* 23, pp. 469-487.

Strecher, V. J., Seijts, G. H., Kok, G., Latham, G. P., Glasgow, R., DeVellis, B., Meertens, R. M. and Bulger, D. W. (1995) 'Goal setting as a strategy for health behavior change', *Health Education Quarterly* 22, pp. 190-200.

Vlahov, D. and Junge, B. (1998) The role of needle exchange programs in HIV prevention *Public Health Reports; 113 (suppl. 1),* pp. 75-80.

17 Stress in the Workplace: A Risk Assessment Approach to Reduction of Risk

REBECCA J. LANCASTER AND ELIZABETH BURTNEY

Abstract

Mental ill health in the workplace is estimated to cost UK employers £6.2 billion each year in lost working days. This is of concern to employers and employees alike, recently highlighted by the HEBS needs assessment study of workplace health promotion, which identified stress as a major issue.

A Health and Safety Executive review (1993) of the stress literature proposed the incorporation of stress within the framework of the assessment and control cycle already introduced to minimise physical health and safety risks. This was supported by the HEBS study that identified health and safety as the predominant health-related culture within Scottish workplaces. It is therefore appropriate to include stress control with other health and safety issues.

The Institute of Occupational Medicine (IOM) had already developed a risk assessment approach entitled the Organisational Stress Health Audit (OSHA) and the feasibility of this was tested in the pilot study commissioned by HEBS.

The OSHA is a three tiered approach. Stage One identifies the presence or absence of work-related stressors and opportunities for risk reduction. Stage Two focuses on investigating areas of particular concern identified in Stage One. Stage Three involves assessing the extent to which recommendations in Stage One and Two have been implemented and their effectiveness.

A database of known causes of work-related stress was compiled from the scientific literature and this formed the background to the OSHA. The OSHA is centred on semi-structured interviews with representatives of all levels and functions within the organisation. The line of questioning follows those known causes of work-related stress in the database.

This paper presents the background to this organisational approach, its feasibility in controlling stress across different types of organisations and future plans for development of the approach.

The views presented are those of the researchers and not the commissioning body.

Introduction

The Health Education Board for Scotland (HEBS) was established in April 1991 as a national agency for health education in Scotland. This health education role is set within the broader context of health promotion which has been defined by the World Health Organisation (WHO) as the process of enabling people to increase control over, and to improve their health (HEBS, 1997).

The health promotion activity of HEBS is delivered through a range of settings that include schools, community, the health service, the general public, voluntary organisations and the workplace. The workplace has been acknowledged as an important arena for health promotion work, given that we can spend up one third of our lives in formal paid work. Thus for those in work can be social environment. It can be viewed as a social and learning environment that may provide an important source of social support and certainly lends itself to promotion work that extends beyond the workplace into the community. (Crosswaite and Jones 1994)

Why Promote Mental Health in the Workplace?

This paper will outline four main reasons, which will highlight the need for mental health promotion in the workplace. First, the broad policy context within which we operate has an influence on our work, particularly Scottish developments. Second, research findings, specifically from research carried out by HEBS indicate the salience of mental health issues in the workplace particularly relating to stress. Third, the high cost of mental health problems to both society and industry, fourth and finally the impending legal responsibilities which employers may soon face.

Mental health has been highlighted as a priority area for a number of years now. However, the focus in the past has mainly been on suicide prevention, at the very extreme end of the spectrum. In Scotland, policy has progressed to the point where the recent green paper for health *Working together for a healthier Scotland* (1998) emphasised the need to prevent mental health problems more generally in addition to promotion of positive mental health. The commitment to this is highlighted in the availability of resources to advance the evidence base for primary, secondary and tertiary prevention.

At the practitioner level, the Scottish Needs Assessment Programme (SNAP, 1994) produced guidance for mental health promotion, a section of which was devoted to mental health promotion in the workplace. This was an important development since this group involves experts in the field of mental health and serves to inform practitioners across Scotland.

A needs assessment was carried out by HEBS (1994) with employees and employers from a range of organisations across Scotland. The participants were asked to discuss their understanding of workplace health promotion, suggest the kind of promotion that would be suitable to their place of employment and determine whose responsibility this might be. The issue of stress was raised spontaneously by employees more than any other health related issue. Sources of stress were identified as workload, job insecurity, poor management and often poor communication between management and employees. These wider issues were of more concern than specific demands from individual work tasks. It was felt that health promotion had a role to play in the reduction of workplace stress.

Published information regarding the costs of mental health problems to the economy varies widely due to the difficulties associated with measuring the problem. For example, based on figures released by the Department of Social Services, it has been estimated that in 1991 mental health problems cost UK industry around £6,200 million (Thompson, 1993). However, the Institute of Management arrived at much higher estimates. They proposed that stress alone was costing the British economy around £7 billion in lost earnings per year (Institute of Management, 1996). If anything, these are underestimates given the stigma associated with reporting stress as a reason for absence.

Employers are increasingly becoming aware of the need to protect mental as well as physical well-being in the workplace. The UK Health and Safety at Work Act of 1974 primarily offers protection to employees at their place of work. In the past this act has been used mainly to deal with physical health. However this now includes stress at work under the guise of 'psychological health'. More recently the Management of Health and Safety at Work Regulations (1992) highlights the need for employers to inform their employees of any risks to health, and this includes mental health.

This is becoming a real concern for employers given the litigation between Walker and Northumberland County Council (1994), a legal case in which a member of staff of the council received compensation for a repeat nervous breakdown.

Approaches to Stress Reduction in the Workplace

There are three main approaches to reducing stress in the workplace: primary; secondary and tertiary.

The primary prevention approach is concerned with identifying and controlling sources of stress in the workplace rather than dealing with an individual's symptoms. This has been called the "risk assessment and hazard control" approach because of its link with the control approach to the management of hazardous substances as outlined in the Control of Substances Hazardous to Health [COSHH] (1988). This approach adopts six steps (commonly known as the control cycle) to reduce the risk of exposure:

1. Identification of the hazard
2. Assessment of the associated risk
3. Implementation of appropriate control strategies
4. Monitoring of effectiveness of control strategies
5. Re-assessment of risk
6. Review of information and training needs of workers exposed to hazards.

This cycle can be applied equally to stress management. Indeed a recent HSE publication recognised identifying and controlling sources of stress in organisations rather than individual-orientated approaches as being the most appropriate, proposing that such investigations should be incorporated into the framework of the assessment and control cycle approach already introduces to minimise physical health and safety risks (Stress at Work – A guide for employers, HSE, 1995).

Secondary prevention is aimed at providing advice and information to enable employees to cope more effectively with stress in their workplace. This is mostly provided in the form of stress management training that helps people understand the causes of stress and how they can help themselves in reducing the impact of the stressors. Health promotion can also be offered and provides an effective channel to inform employees of the importance of good diet, physical exercise, relaxation in the management of stress, both work-related and from other sources.

Tertiary prevention focuses on individual employees who are suffering

158

from stress. Schemes such as the Employee Assistance Programme (EAP) can be introduced into a company, which provide counselling for the employee. However this approach, while useful for the individual employee, is limited in that the organisation itself gets very little feedback regarding the nature and causes of the problems. The symptoms of stress rather than the sources of stress are dealt with through tertiary prevention.

The Organisational Stress Health Audit (OSHA)

The OSHA is a cross-functional, top down, primary intervention acting at the organisational level. Therefore, the approach sought to ensure that staff at all levels within the organisation were represented, and included as many different disciplines as possible. It is also consistent with the risk management control cycle framework adopted for most other health and safety hazards. The OSHA is a three-stage approach to stress management at source, with hazard identification, risk assessment, review of existing control measures, recommendations for improved control, and evaluation of control all embodied in it. The aim of Stage I of the OSHA is to provide an organisational overview by identifying the presence or absence of work-related stressors and opportunities for risk reduction. Stage II focuses on investigating in more detail areas of concern identified in Stage I, e.g. a group of employees operating under particularly high pressure, or a specific issue such as communication of change. Stage III involves assessing the extent to which actions identified in Stages I and II have been implemented and their effectiveness in reducing organisational stress.

Outline of Study Design

Given the weight of evidence in favour of the primary prevention approach to stress reduction in the workplace it seemed appropriate for HEBS to invest in the development of this method. In 1996, HEBS commissioned the IOM to assess the feasibility in terms of cost and acceptability of applying the OSHA in Scottish workplaces. The aims of the project were as follows:

1. To recruit two to three organisations to participate in the pilot project.
2. To work with all levels and interest groups within the organisations in order to assess the feasibility of developing the risk assessment and haz-

ard control approach.

3. To evaluate and fully document the processes involved in recruiting participating organisations and in identifying and implementing the organisational changes required.
4. To pilot methods for evaluating the impact and outcomes of the risk assessment and hazard control approach.
5. To produce detailed recommendations about appropriate ways of developing and implementing the approach.

In this study, Stages I and II of the OSHA were applied in three organisations. Each company appointed a co-ordinator to assist with recruitment of personnel and scheduling the work. The company contact also provided background information about the organisations' organisational structure, policies, processes, pattern of workforce, sickness absence/staff turnover and health and safety issues. The co-ordinator was also part of a steering group, comprising representatives of senior management, line managers and employee representatives, established to ensure that all parties were aware of the study and were able to contribute to the work programme. The Company contact used various methods to recruit participants, i.e. personal contact, e-mail and cascade/team briefings, each having advantages and disadvantages.

The background information, provided by the company contact, was used in the development of semi-structured interview questionnaires for Stage I. Each questionnaire was tailored to the position, function and likely knowledge/ experience of the individual to be interviewed, and also took account of relevant issues within the company. The interview questionnaires were designed to identify potential stressors, characterised as Environmental (organisation's structure, work characteristics, policies), Physical (work characteristics, policies) and Psychosocial (human resource management, individual factors, management structure). Interviewees were selected to ensure that each level and department was represented, from Senior Management down. The interviews were conducted by IOM Occupational Psychologists and an Occupational Physician, as appropriate, and recorded on audio tapes. These tapes were transcribed, and the information collated and summarised by the interviewers. This was then discussed by an IOM multi-disciplinary team, a procedure which provided a comprehensive overview of the results and facilitated the production of a confidential written report for each company (a specimen report is included as an Appendix). Each report was also presented and discussed at a feedback meeting, together with recommendations for Stage II.

In Stage II, the investigation conducted in each organisation was one where it was considered that intervention could have helped in the short term.

In two of the companies, the focus was on a specific group of employees highlighted from Stage I as being under particularly high pressure due to issues of workload, staffing levels or job design. In these cases, semi-structured questionnaires were developed by IOM following a process meeting with representatives of the focus group. These formed the basis of interviews (conducted by the same interviewers as in Stage I) with individuals from this group, together with others who interacted with them. These personnel also completed three self-administered standard questionnaires i.e. the General Health Questionnaire (GHQ-12), the Stress Anxiety Questionnaire (SAQ) and the Work Environment Scale (WES). In the third company, Stage I had identified poor communication of change as an important stressor, so the Stage II investigation focused on examining the potential for improvements by means of an attitudinal survey. This involved several employee groups completing a self-administered questionnaire, developed by the IOM for this study, and a Team Climate Inventory, to assess team working and potential sources of resistance to change.

All results in Stage II were analysed with reference to data provided by the designers of each standard questionnaire and/or data obtained for comparison employee groups within the organisation. As with Stage I, confidential written reports were provided to each company, but no feed-back presentations were made because of time constraints. Summary findings of the Stage II investigations are presented in an Appendix.

After each Stage, questionnaires were distributed to company contacts and participants to canvass their views on the OSHA approach.

Main Outcomes

The main outcomes in relation to the six objectives are summarised as follows:

1. Recruitment of Companies

The companies recruited represent both public and private sectors, and industrial and service sectors. They varied in size and complexity, from those employing several hundred to several thousand, and operating from one to several sites. Within each, there was a diversity of function and age ranges represented. The organisations had variously experienced upsizing, downsizing and restructuring, with consequent differences in uncertainty over future em-

161

ployment. The relative importance of specific health and safety issues also varied across the organisations.

The organisations which took part in the study were existing contacts of the IOM or HEBS who had expressed concerns about stress. Methods of recruiting organisations to adopt such an approach were therefore limited.

2. Cross-functional, Top-down Approach

The study demonstrated that it was, in practice, possible to ensure a cross-functional and top-down approach for each of the companies taking part. Involvement of senior management in the interview process ensured commitment from the top to the whole exercise and comprehensive coverage of all aspects of organisational policies and procedures. The use of company contacts generally facilitated the recruitment of personnel, ensured the smooth running of the investigations, and maintained feedback on progress within the organisation. The commitment of the company contact was a significant factor in determining the rate of progress of the investigations. The use of a systematic approach (based upon an organisational chart for the company involved, the need to ensure that all sectors of the company were represented, and the use of skilled interviewers) minimised the potential for selection bias by contacts or senior staff within the organisation. The benefits of holding process meetings prior to commencement of Stage I, and involving more employees at this stage, became increasingly apparent as the study progressed.

3. Risk Assessment/Management Approach to Organisational Stress

Risk assessment/management strategies are applied to most other occupational health and safety hazards, and it was felt that companies would be familiar with this approach, and address the hazard of occupational stress more appropriately. The feedback from company contacts and other personnel within the companies suggests that the two Stages of the OSHA that were conducted were effective in identifying organisational stressors, areas/groups at high risk and recommendations for risk reduction. General themes were identified as common to all three organisations and these were: workload and pressures to deliver services; uncertainty about the future in relation to job security; lack of resources (financial/staffing); and poor communication or lack of consultation on relevant issues. Companies showed a willingness to implement recommendations, but the extent to which these were implemented and the opportunity to evaluate their impact were limited by the restricted timescale of the study.

4. Evaluation and Documentation of the Process

The response from companies clearly indicated that the approach has benefits in terms of effectiveness, minimal down-time and disruption, and limited costs of the process. The OSHA has also proved to be flexible across industry sectors; across different circumstances of change; and within individual companies where interviews or questionnaires could be modified to address specific factors.

Information on potential occupational stressors collected during Stage II was found to support that collected in Stage I, despite different tools or techniques being used in each Stage; different groups within the organisation being assessed; and different individuals being involved, thus providing a degree of validation of the methodology.

5. Pilot Methods for Evaluating Impact and Outcomes of the Approach

Companies were taking steps to implement specific recommendations e.g. review of policies or procedures, changes in work design, or improving sickness absence monitoring. Evaluation of the impact and outcomes of the recommendations made, however, was limited by the time constraints of the project. This is an objective of Stage III of the OSHA. However the process was evaluated by sending questionnaires to participants and company contacts. The information collected included assessments of the usefulness and appropriateness of the methodology in identifying relevant sources of occupational stress, the time and resources required by the organisation, and the quality of the information provided by the IOM. For the two Stages of the OSHA which were completed, the response from companies, as to their benefits, was positive.

6. Development and Implementation of the Approach

At present, the effective application of the OSHA depends on accurate data collection and analysis by interviewers trained in relevant disciplines such as psychology. Standard structured interview shells were produced, but the detailed content was modified for each organisation and also during the interview schedule. This was possible due to the interpretive skills of the trained interviewers. This inherent flexibility allowed emerging issues to be fully explored and is a vital element in the success of the approach. Other important elements include the multi-disciplinary team approach and its independence, both in analysing the data which is collected and in providing recommendations for further investigation, or for risk reduction, which are appropriate and practical for the particular company.

Conclusions

The main aim of this pilot project was to assess the feasibility, in terms of cost and acceptability, of developing the risk assessment/hazard control approach to workplace stress in Scottish workplaces, with emphasis on the private sector. This study has clearly demonstrated the feasibility of Stages I and II of the OSHA in identifying a range of work - related stressors across different organisations. Companies showed a willingness to implement recommendations made on risk reduction measures. A second aim of the study was to provide a basis for developing a larger scale controlled trial of the approach. This project has identified a number of aspects which could be incorporated in such a study, including:

- conducting Stage III in the companies which participated in this pilot study to assess to what extent recommendations from Stages I and II have been implemented and their impact, and identifying new stressors (if any);
- extending coverage to more companies to increase the range of systems and practices identified as being beneficial in reducing levels of organisational stress and related factors, thereby developing a database of good practice which could assist other organisations nationally;
- assessing the feasibility of applying Stage II, either alone or followed by Stage I and/or III, in situations where companies have already identified high risk groups;
- evaluating the effectiveness of different methods of recruitment;
- developing and validating tools/techniques which could be applied by organisations themselves (including small companies), particularly those with limited knowledge of occupational stress. These could include a checklist to aid identification of workplace stressors, and improved software packages for recording and monitoring sickness absence data and which are flexible enough to be used across a range of industries. These,

together with 'good practice' risk reduction measures and other information, could be used to improve guidance and training for management, supervisors and other employees.

It is concluded that the OSHA is effective in identifying potential causes of stress and generating recommendations for risk reduction in both public and private sector organisations. Planned further work will be instrumental in evaluating and monitoring this approach to establish its effectiveness in reducing the causes of stress in organisations at source and subsequently reducing symptoms of work related stress among employees.

References

Crosswaite, C. and Jones, L. (1994) *Workplace health promotion: a literature review Scotland and the UK*, Health Education Board for Scotland.

HSC (1992) Management of Health and Safety at Work Regulations, Approved Code of Practice, HMSO Publications, London.

Institute of Management (1996) *Are Managers Under Stress?* Institute of Management, London.

Jones, L. and Ross, A. (1994) *Health Promotion in the Workplace. Needs Assessment Research Project,* Health Education Board for Scotland, Edinburgh.

Scottish Needs Assessment Programme (1994). *Mental Health Overview and Programme,* Scottish Forum for Public Health Medicine.

The Scottish Office (1998) *Working together for a healthier Scotland*, The Scottish Office, Edinburgh.

Thompson, D. (1993) *Mental Illness: the Fundamental Facts*, Mental Health Foundation, London.

18 Developing Strategic Partnerships

ROS LOBO AND CHRIS GILLEARD

Abstract

The Mental Health Promotion Alliance for Merton Sutton and Wandsworth has been working to establish a positive mental health strategy for all three boroughs included in the MSW Health Authority's catchment area. The task for the Alliance is to work with various organisations and groups in the three boroughs to facilitate a broad brush strategy that can establish mental health promotion as a central component of a "health action initiative".

Much of our effort focuses upon developing programmes that increase the resilience of individuals, groups and communities and reduce those 'noxious' features that impair or jeopardise mental health. To do this we plan to work systemically with seven key institutional structures: *education*, *employment*, the *environment*, *health*, *housing*, *leisure* and the *media.*

The broad outline of this programme first was outlined in a "pre-strategy statement" - a message of intent which has received the support from all three borough focused Mental Health Strategy groups in Merton, Sutton and Wandsworth, as well as the broad support of the Health Authority and the three Local Authorities. Putting flesh on this statement of intent is the task of five key working groups we have set up, targeting one or other of the institutional structures in the pre-strategy statement [health, education, employment, environment and leisure, and the media]. The work of these groups will be described to illustrate one way of "selling" mental health promotion.

Introduction

The Merton Sutton and Wandsworth Mental Health Promotion Alliance was established in 1995 as an association linking the local health authority with mental health service providers, local authority representatives and local non-statutory services sharing a common agenda to help promote the mental health of the local population.

In January 1997 a 'pre-strategy statement' was produced that outlined a framework for developing mental health promotion as a partnership with local employers, local authorities and local communities. The focus was on the promotion of positive mental health for the community, for families within the community and for individuals themselves. We identified four main age groups, and six principal institutional structures. Our age groups were - infants/ pre-school children; school/college age children and adolescents; adults; and older adults. Our key institutional structures were - education, employment, environment [include. housing], health, leisure and the media.

We presented this 'statement of intent' to the three borough focused mental health strategy groups and to the local health authority and the three local government authorities. In broad terms the statement has been approved by all these bodies. Mental health promotion is now part of the development plans of the Health Authority. Now we are facing the task of delivering a concrete programme that can win local support and prove of measurable benefit to the local community.

Where to Begin?

On October 10th 1997 [World Mental Health Day] we launched our statement of intent to develop a mental health promotion strategy for the three local boroughs of Merton Sutton and Wandsworth. During the seminar which served as the launch we distributed four leaflets outlining a] our overall message of promoting positive mental health; b] information about mental health and the environment; c] information about mental health, stress and the workplace and d] the results of a survey of mental health promotional resources we had found in local Primary Care services.

Arising directly from that seminar we developed four mental health promotion 'working groups' focusing upon one or other of the institutional structures that we viewed as key to developing appropriate strategic partnerships. The four groups were:

- Mental health and education group
- Mental health and work group
- Mental health, leisure and the environment group
- Mental health promotion in primary health care.

The Programme

Each group is made up of a small core of 'volunteer members', whose main task is to make contact with key groups and figures to establish a wider network within which to develop a strategic programme for each structure/group. The objectives for these networks are:

- collate and distribute information relevant to mental health promotion,
- propose and 'sponsor' particular projects designed as active interventions to prevent/make less likely mental health problems in either vulnerable groups or host communities,
- increase awareness of mental health as an issue touching everyone - in all spheres of life.

Members of these groups are also linking up to other existing structures and contributing to other linked programmes. Each group reports back to the Mental Health Promotion Alliance on progress. On World Mental Health Day, October 10th 1999 we aim to convene a programme to celebrate the achievements that have been made, identify the tasks lie ahead, and establish the objectives that need to be set for the new 'millennium'.

The work done by these groups will be considered later in this paper.

Links with Local Government

A key task for the Alliance is to work together with all three local authorities to help draw out links between civic strategies and the aims of mental health promotion. Useful links are beginning to be forged with Merton Sutton and Wandsworth Borough Councils but these links are slow to develop and require considerable caution given the very different political stances of each borough [Labour, Liberal Democrat and Conservative led respectively]. Nevertheless we are hopeful that these links will help drive the strategy forward into concrete programmes that incorporate a mental health promotion perspective.

The main links established so far include proposals for 50 mental health promotion projects put forward to one of the boroughs, Wandsworth. Of these 50 proposals, 21 are being taken through the borough's Policy and Planning Unit by the senior health policy analyst who himself is a member of the Alliance. They also are being considered within the developing Health Improvement Programme being established by the Health Authority. Some of these 21 proposals are outlined over the page [full details of the proposals are available separately from the authors].

Our next steps include inviting local politicians to the MHP Alliance meetings, arranging presentations to various groups within each Borough [i.e. Leisure, Housing, Social Services, Environmental Services] to raise awareness of the scope for MHP work. One illustration of this 'political' dimension is the news release of one of the local Sutton MPs drawing attention to the forthcoming World Mental Heath Day and the work of the Alliance. Another was the involvement of the Mayor of Merton in chairing a meeting on Depression and Asian Women during National Depression Week.

The Work of the MHP Sub-Groups

1. Mental Health Promotion and the Work Place

The sub-group dealing with work has focused upon [a] accessing the literature on work related stress and [b] developing links with the three local Chambers of Commerce, informing them of the importance of the work place for mental health. We have built up a reasonable literature in the area of work related stress and this has provided the information to produce a leaflet for employers concerning "Work and Well-being".

We continue to develop our contacts with the local business community. One preliminary meeting took place earlier this year, and we hope to continue strengthening our links, with further meetings and presentations. It is gratifying that some local employers are now making use of Specialist Health Promotion resources to improve their own understanding of the relevance of mental health issues at work.

We are working with the three Chambers of Commerce to gather information about the views of local employers toward stress and the workplace. We have developed a questionnaire to gather this information in a systematic form. This will provide the basis in working out a more focused

Figure 1: Illustrative projects proposed by the Alliance to Wandsworth Borough Council

1. **Mental fitness classes in leisure centres:** offering stress control, massage, relaxation and meditation/yoga: employing p/t 'mental fitness trainer for one year as a pilot and judge take-up and satisfaction.

2. **Self-help leaflets, videos audiotapes and books in public libraries:** ensuring that local libraries have a wide range of resources for people to 'cope' with anxiety, depression and related problems, and promoting awareness through 'themed' weeks or fortnights, including talks and other presentations.

3. **Saturday Clubs for vulnerable children about to move to secondary school:** lack of social networks and poor self-esteem/confidence place children at risk of being bullied and developing emotional disorders. Volunteer led Saturday Clubs during the last year of Primary School and the summer holiday before Secondary School starts would aim to build social and physical self-confidence [trainee teachers/school counsellors and youth workers could take part].

4. **"After school" schools for young people:** develop a network across selected secondary schools in the borough so that young people can if they wish return to their old school for get togethers/socials/sport etc. over the week-ends or during holidays. Aim to reduce the potential difficulties between leaving school and work - especially for those not going on to further education.

5. **Pre-retirement courses for all over 45s in local Adult Colleges:** places to be sponsored by local employers and training input provided from local sources of expertise such as police and security: pensions officers and welfare rights: financial advisors and pensions/general financial advice.

6. **Family Centre for parents with alcohol problems:** Seek local support to set up a drop in centre for families where one or both parents have an alcohol problem, providing an informal setting in the afternoons and early evening where CAB staff, alcohol counsellors and child support workers would be accessible and where a non medicalised system focusing upon family support could help families facing the disruption arising from alcohol abuse.

7. **Developing mental health training programmes for housing officers:** Look at the experiences of people working at the front end of the Housing Department and build on existing training programmes to develop an awareness of mental health and mental ill health and housing issues that is not confined to the tasks of housing people with serious mental illness.

local strategy to involve employers in an active campaign to address mental health stress and the workplace.

2. Mental Health, Well-being and Education

The sub-group on well-being and education has adopted a similar approach - of gathering relevant literature and of developing links with the local education authorities. We have gathered information about topics such as bullying, building self-esteem, emotional literacy and examples of curriculum based programmes on mental health that fit within the stream of PSE (Personal and Social Education, now expanded to include Personal, Social and Health Education).

This information was used to produce a second leaflet called "Education and Well-being", developed in collaboration with the PSE and Healthy Schools co-ordinator and Young Persons Programme Manager. This leaflet has been distributed to all local schools in Merton Sutton and Wandsworth and the three Directors of Education.

We have not neglected the area of adult education. Discussions have taken place about expanding the curricula of the local adult education colleges to incorporate courses with relevance to promoting mental health. Our aim is to set up a number of such courses that can provide a range of mental health relevant skills - ranging from life skills classes to managing stress and managing change.

We have had one preliminary meeting with staff from local primary schools. Out of this meeting we are planning to collect useful resources for teachers, special needs teachers particularly and for teachers' aides and school nurses to help staff identify agencies and other resources to handle difficulties presented by children at school. In addition the meeting was helpful in shaping the contents and format of a questionnaire that is being developed to identify the issues necessary before developing a local strategy to promote mental health and well-being in schools. Thirdly the issue of stress upon teachers arose from this meeting. We plan to look at ways of helping teachers in inner city areas cope with problems of violence, abuse and difficult to control youngsters without resorting to exclusion. Finally the topic of working in partnership with parents was raised and the difficulties that can sometimes arise out of the seeming lack of interest or even hostility that teachers can feel from the parents.

It is clear that teachers themselves feel uncertain about the limits of their own role - and how far their 'pastoral' responsibilities extend in addressing the 'non-educational' needs of the children in their charge. This in turn raises issues about teacher training and the extent to which teachers feel competent in fulfilling such 'health promoting' tasks. We plan to convene more meetings to discuss these issues once the results of our survey of local schools is completed. At present we are still piloting the questionnaire for use with local schools and hope to begin the survey proper in November '98. Once the results are in we will set up meetings in each of the three boroughs to share our findings and focus our strategy, working also with local child and adolescent mental health services.

Increasingly it is becoming evident that there need to be links between schools, local child and adolescent mental health services and local authorities. Mental health promotion is moving up the agenda within the proposed National Services Framework for Mental Health. We will be working with the Health Authority to formulate plans to engage both local schools and local services in the development of mental health promotion programmes for school age children across the three boroughs.

3. Mental Health and the Environment

Prior to setting up this subgroup we had already done some literature research and prepared a leaflet on mental health and the environment that was distributed on World Mental Health Day, October '97. We have made links with local environmental services, the Police and their Vulnerable Persons' Unit, local Directors of Housing and Leisure, local Agenda 21 initiatives and local Community Development Workers.

A preliminary meeting was held with the Community Development Workers and local Environmental Services. They were able to give us information about local development projects and how we could access these projects. Community development workers in turn can become the links between mental health promotion and urban regeneration programmes. One outcome of this meeting was that three of the community development workers took on such an active role.

In Sutton, as a consequence, one of the Sutton based community development workers was able to secure a grant from the HEA for the Sutton Mental Health Promotion Group [an association affiliated with MSW Mental Health Promotion Alliance] World Mental Health Day campaign this October.

Further, we have been able to feed in to the participatory needs assessment that is being carried out as part of the Single Regeneration Budget programme for the northern wards in Sutton by including mental health promotion within their agenda and the importance of early intervention and prevention in addressing mental health problems.

In Merton, two proposals have been made, via the community

development workers in partnership with MSW Mental Health Promotion Alliance, for funding increased creche facilities and a support worker for single mothers. This bid followed a seminar on single mothers that was held in one of the local schools in June this year. The bid was made to Merton Council and appears to have been successful. We look forward to working together on this project. A second bid followed National Depression Week, in April this year. A seminar was held to look at depression amongst Asian women in Merton. Out of this seminar, a group of Asian women established a management committee/network to raise awareness and look at how they can influence policy and local service provision to improve the mental health of their community.

Also in Merton, we were advised to put in a bid for funds as part of a general SRB project, specifically to identify 'vulnerable groups' registered with local GP practices and develop a 'primary care based' mental health promotion programme with two local practices, with a total population of approximately 12,000 people. The bid is for an initial three year period with scope for further development for five more years. At present we still await the outcome of this bid . This will be elaborated further when we discuss the work of the primary care group.

In Wandsworth we are working with the Ethnic Minority Linkworker/ Co-ordinator to establish a similar forum to address mental health issues within the Asian communities using the forthcoming World Mental Health Day as a focus for the campaign.

4. Mental Health Promotion in Primary Care

A sub-group for promoting mental health in primary care has met regularly since February. Three projects are currently being undertaken. The first was the development and distribution of a Mental Health Resources Directory for Primary Care. This directory was developed from previous work based on the Health in Mind project conducted during 1996/97. The Health in Mind project was our first venture into providing a mental health promotion servicve within primary care and several useful lessons arose from this [Brown et al., 1997; Gilleard and Lobo, 1998]. We outlined the HiM project at the International Conference on Mental Health Promotion , held at Troon, last year. Copies of the directory were finally published in June this year have been sent to all GP surgeries throughout Merton Sutton and Wandsworth. Already we have had useful feedback from a number of GP s, and we shall continue to seek quarterly feedback reports and produce updates as necessary.

Secondly we produced a paper for the group reviewing mental health and vulnerability for the primary care team. This in turn has led to a proposal for the establishment of a Risk Profiling Project for Mental Health in Primary Care. This project is linked with the University of London's Queen Mary and Westfield College. Joint funding has now been agreed from the Department of Health, the Regional Executive, the local Health Authority and the local Mental Health Services Trust to carry out a three year piece of work targeting three practice populations in Merton Sutton and Wandsworth. The third piece of work is the production of a leaflet outlining the need for mental health promotion in primary care and is intended for all members of the PHCT. It is currently in draft form and we hope to send out a final version for World Mental Health Day.

Finally the work of the Primary Care subgroup has received recognition from the Regional executive when we were invited to attend a workshop on Mental Health and Primary Care Groups. At this workshop we were able to discuss the scope for mental health promotion within the Primary Care setting. We introduced the idea of a needs based methodology for mental health promotion within the PC setting and the importance of a commissioning strategy to make mental health promotion a key part of any PCG commission for mental health services. The work of the Alliance has also been recognised in the national database for mental health innovations in Primary Care, established by the Sainsbury Trust and commissioned by the NHS Executive. Locally the newly released Primary Care Development Plan for Wandsworth [1998-2003] has explicitly included the work of the Alliance and its role in developing a strategy for Primary Care based Mental Health Promotion.

Discussion and Conclusions

The work of the MSW Mental Health Promotion Alliance continues to grow and extend its involvement with a variety of local services, resources and communities. Recognition of our work has come from the Mental Health team of the Health Education Authority. The work of the Alliance and our outline strategy are included as a case study in developing a local strategy for mental health promotion in the forthcoming HEA publication "Community Action for Mental Health", which is being published as one of the HEA's key resources for this year's World Mental Health Day campaign [HEA, 1998].

Within the local health economy the work of the Alliance is growing. We have been invited by the Health Authority to submit plans for mental health promotion for the next two years. We hope that we shall gain further ideas from this conference in preparing our short term strategic plans.

175

Our message for the conference is this. Mental health promotion is growing in importance. The MSW Mental Health Promotion Alliance has succeeded in placing its strategy on the agenda of all three local authorities' Mental Health Strategy groups, on the Primary Care Development Plans for the next five years, and has gained support from local politicians. We are forming closer links with schools, colleges, local employers and local primary care services, with local authorities and of course our local Health Authority. We are collating information and conducting research to increase our knowledge of what has been done, what can be done and what is wanted in the area of mental health promotion. We are working both to promote positive mental health and to prevent mental ill-health; at both a population level, and at targeted populations.

When the MSW Mental Health Promotion Alliance was first formed, it was a lone voice coming from a very few interested persons. Our voice has grown louder and an increasing number of institutions are beginning to listen and take seriously the prospect that we can improve the mental health of our community.

References

Brown M., Gilleard C. and Lobo R. (1997) Health in Mind: A Mental Health Promotion Service in Primary Care. Evaluation Report, *Merton Sutton and Wandsworth Health Authority, Dept of Public Health, London.*

Gilleard C. and Lobo R. (1998) 'Attendees at a primary care based mental health promotion drop-in clinic', *Psychiatric Bulletin* vol. 22, pp. 559-562.

Health Education Authority (1998) 'Developing a local strategy for mental health promotion: a case study.' In *Community action for Mental Health*, HEA, London, pp.7-13.

19 Comparing Paradigms in Mental Health Promotion Evaluation and Research

GLENN MACDONALD

Abstract

The paper contends that a vital aspect of the evaluation of mental health promotion concerns the way in which 'mental health' is being conceptualised and operationalised in the intervention. Further, just as there are different and competing 'theories of the problem' of mental health promotion, then also, there are differences in how mental health promotion can or should be researched or evaluated. These differences are not merely of opinion or point of view but emerge from different assumptions about the nature of knowledge, how it is generated and how it can be investigated. Drawing on work from Labonte and Robertson (1996), the paper explores the details and assumptions of two competing epistemologies – the positivist and the social constructionist – which are seen as driving both research and practice. Included in this analysis are a number of research issues such as the acceptability of single or multiple accounts of reality and the purpose of the research. Questions are also raised about the assumed value or status of research from the two competing traditions. In particular, the belief that the method of evaluation somehow adds credibility to the practice or intervention being evaluated is challenged. Finally, issues about acknowledging various stages of intervention evaluation are explored with special reference to a conceptual distinction between impact and outcome. Some implications for how mental health promotion can be evaluated or researched are identified.

Introduction

This paper sets out to examine the implications for researching and evaluating mental health promotion of the judgement that mental health promotion, and health promotion more generally are contested areas of intervention whose practice can often be seen to fall into fairly distinct and frequently competing or opposing approaches. As early as 1985, Ewles and Simnet mapped out a five-approach analysis of health promotion claiming a differentiation between medical, behaviour change, educational, client centred, and social change approaches. Although this analysis can be criticised, it does show significant differences in the way that some of these approaches theorise the problem and promote a solution. The slightly later work of French and Adams (1986) also identifies significant differences in terms of the ethics and effectiveness of competing health promotion approaches. Other work has identified fundamental differences between health promotion approaches at an epistemological and ideological level (Caplan and Holland, 1990), and this analysis has been applied to mental health promotion (Tudor 1992, 1996; MacDonald 1993).

The paper contends that these different ways of theorising the problem and of identifying solutions are not only evident in health promotion practice, but are also relevant in terms of how such practice is researched or evaluated. This is because as researchers or evaluators, we are not immune from making similar epistemological and ideological assumptions. Clarity is needed both in terms of the focus or object of the research and also its process. That is, research about mental health needs to aim for

- a *conceptual* understanding of the fundamental differences involved in intervention approaches being researched (i.e. a conceptual understanding of the objects of the research),
- a *reflexive* understanding of these fundamental differences which are also involved in research or evaluation approaches (i.e. a reflexive understanding of the process of the research).

Although the paper is written specifically with mental health promotion in mind, I would argue that its content is also significant for health promotion more generally.

A Conceptual Basis for Mental Health Promotion - What is it we are Researching?

Clearly there has been major contention about the concept of mental health. Any approach to the promotion of mental health will relate to the view taken about the nature of mental health. And how mental health promotion is researched and evaluated will also be dependant upon the view taken about the nature of mental health. The SHEPS Position Paper on Mental Health Promotion : **"Ten Elements of Mental Health, its Promotion and Demotion"** (MacDonald and O'Hara, 1996), identifies ten elements of mental health and argues that such a wide-ranging and complex concept cannot be addressed in simplistic ways.. These can be summarised as follows:

According to this map, mental health can be promoted by increasing or enhancing the elements above the dotted line, and by decreasing or diminishing the elements below it. Several strengths have been claimed for this map that cannot be rehearsed here. The main point here is that in any research or evaluation needs to identify its area of concern and further, which particular conceptualisation of mental health is being identified or assumed in the intervention. This is not a neutral or irrelevant choice – clearly how 'mental

Figure 1: A Map of Elements of Mental Health, its Promotion and Demotion

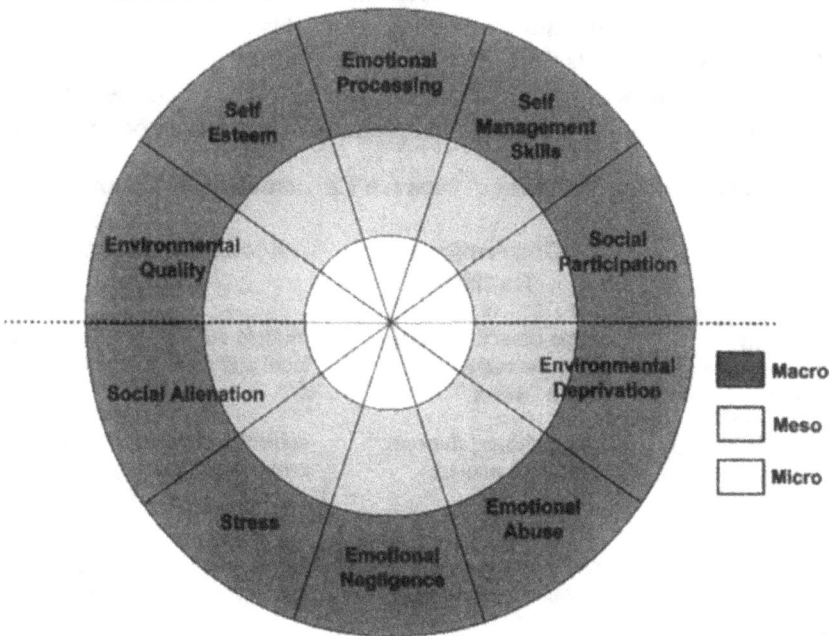

179

health' is being theorised within an intervention has deep implications for how effective the intervention is likely to be. This point is returned to below.

So in researching or evaluating mental health promotion, it needs to be made clear which element or elements of mental health are being specifically addressed, so that the evaluation method can be seen to be appropriate to the aim of the intervention. An aim such as "To improve the mental health of ......" is probably too broad and general even for an aim, except perhaps at strategy level. For specific interventions, something more specific - like an objective situated in one of the ten elements with specific reference to the appropriate level(s) (micro, meso and macro) - is probably more realistic. This would contribute to what McLeroy et al (1994) call a clearer and more overt 'theory of the problem'.

A Theoretical Framework for Mental Health Promotion - Assumptions Driving Research and Practice

Fundamental Differences

I have claimed above that how mental health promotion is researched and evaluated will also be dependent upon the view taken about the nature of mental health. In examining the implications of this further, perhaps the first thing to acknowledge is that differences in how mental health is described or characterised, as well as differences in views as to how it can be promoted usually arise out of fairly fundamental philosophical positions on such things

Table 1: Exploring Differences between Epistemological Traditions

	Conventional Tradition	Social Constructionist Tradition
Ontology (assumptions about the nature of reality)	single objective reality universal truths cause - effect	multiple subjective realities local and specific truths
Epistemology (beliefs about what in principle we can know about reality)	subject-object dualism value-free enquiry	subject and object interrelated creation of inquiry process
Methodology (ways of finding out about reality)	hypothesis testing context-free variables	hermeneutic and dialectic interaction and synthesis

as the nature of reality, what we can in principle know about that reality, and what all this implies for ways of finding out about that reality. Labonte and Robertson (1996) claim that in effect, there are two paramount positions or traditions that these assumptions and beliefs fall into - the conventional (or positivist) and the social constructionist (or interpretive, or phenomenological). They have mapped out some of the differences as in table 1.

Following on from this, it would of course be possible to map out the finer detail such as differences like:

- the aim or purpose of the research
- the status of research and of its findings
- how variability is dealt with
- how the trustworthiness of the research is judged
- how generalisable the research findings are judged to be
- what are the ethics of the relationship between researcher and researched.

However, rather than drawing out these differences in detail, my purpose in this paper is to draw out some of the implications for researching or evaluating mental health promotion of following the general assumptions or beliefs of either one paradigm or another. However, at this stage I want to note that using this sort of analysis can be taken further to include other aspects of mental health promotion, for example its epidemiological basis and how 'mental health' has been conceptualised. So, for example, we could argue that in the conventional and constructionist traditions, the following differences emerge:

Table 2: Exploring Health Differences within Epistemological Traditions

	Conventional Tradition	Social Constructionist Tradition
Epidemiology	individual lifestyles behavioural risk factors	social equality relative deprivation risk factors
Concepts of health	pathogenic view of mental ill-health disintegrative, mind-body split	salutogenic view of mental health integrative, holistic

181

It perhaps needs to be added that these categorisations are broad and general. It often appears that actual health promotion practice seems to fall across both categories. But inconsistency between practice and its theoretical base is nothing new and just as in other areas of health promotion, it seems clear that health promotion practitioners and commissioners need to be aware of which philosophical tradition their work it is based on or rooted in, and whether any inconsistencies (e.g., a community involvement approach based on an individual lifestyle epidemiology) are acceptable or problematic. And a very important point here reiterates the issue about how mental health is being conceptualised – clearly, the position taken in the SHEPS ten element map (fig1 above) derives from the salutogenic view.

Conceptual Issues - Important Distinctions in Researching and Evaluating Health Promotion

The fundamental distinctions identified above serve as a backdrop to the issue of research and evaluation in mental health promotion and some detail about this is covered later. Firstly however, I think it is necessary to cover some conceptual ground regarding the nature of health promotion research and evaluation.

The most important conceptual issue to sort out is what counts as effectiveness in health promotion. In considering issues of effectiveness, a useful model shows four points of evaluation : input, process, impact and outcome. More accurately, it is perhaps better to describe what goes on at each of the four stages as an audit. This is because what is being collected ought to be information set against expected or desired criteria such as budgets, quality standards, codes of practice, participation targets, etc. and this is essentially descriptive rather than evaluative. True evaluation comes when making *judgements* about the various items of information collected. So evaluation goes beyond *what* happened and makes some judgement about this.

Overall there are perhaps two types of judgement to be made. Firstly, a project's **technical effectiveness** (after Smee, 1995) can be judged by whether enough of the desired impact results from acceptable processes carried out with well managed inputs. However, such an evaluation will only tell us how well the project performed against the impact objectives and targets that were set. Another form of evaluation, namely **allocative effectiveness** would tell us whether these impact objectives and targets were the right ones to go for in the first place. In other words:

Figure 2: A Model of an Evaluation Process

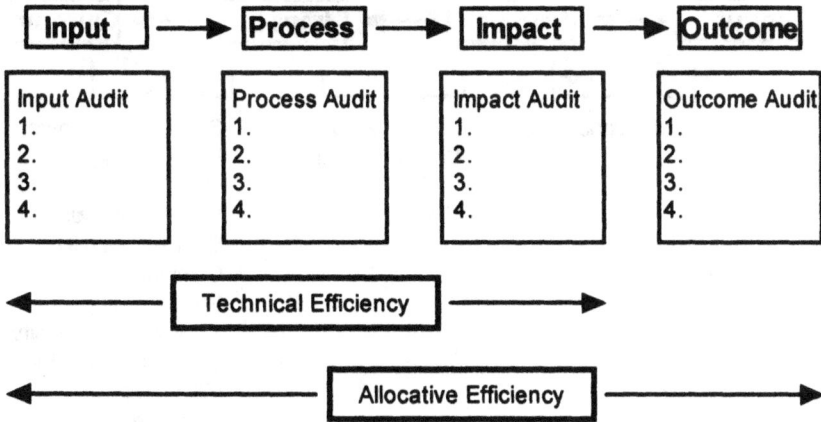

Technical Efficiency = Doing things right
Allocative Efficiency = Doing the right things   Smee (1995)

But in order to make evaluations of either technical or allocative effectiveness, I think we need to make 'sub-evaluations' at the links between each stage. What could be included as such 'sub-evaluations' are shown in the next figure. It seems to me that the most difficult and the most significant questions are those that relate impact to outcome and this is the area where I think health promotion specialists need to be making their mark. What I hope is clear from the figure is that much of this evaluative activity can best be done *prior to* rather than following behind health promotion activity. i.e. *proactive* rather than reactive. Thus we could and should be evaluating *existing* practice and policy, as well as future possibilities. This is an important point because good evaluation of this sort would prevent resources being wasted on activity which is - *in an allocative sense* - never going to be effective nomatter how well it can be carried out.

In many cases of mental health promotion the evaluation seem to me to offer no real distinction between impact and outcome. Or the terms 'impact', 'outcome' and 'output' are used interchangeably. I don't think this will do. An impact of an intervention is the effect it has in the immediate term on those participating in it. An outcome is a longer term and wider measure - the 'impact of the impacts' we might say. With this distinction in mind it is possible to ask whether the **impact of an intervention is on the way to effecting wider, more sustained and general mental health outcomes.** This question

183

Figure 3: Evaluative Factors Between each Evaluation Stage

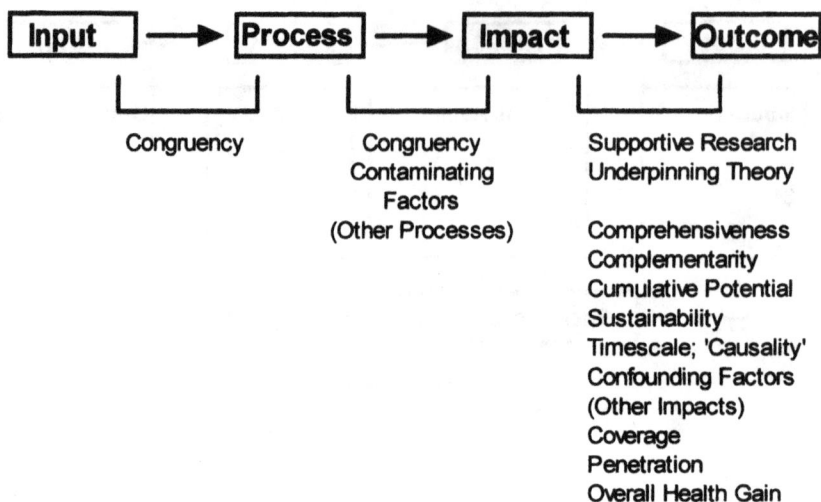

Input	→	Process	→	Impact	→	Outcome

Congruency	Congruency Contaminating Factors (Other Processes)	Supportive Research Underpinning Theory Comprehensiveness Complementarity Cumulative Potential Sustainability Timescale; 'Causality' Confounding Factors (Other Impacts) Coverage Penetration Overall Health Gain

asks about the amount of mental health gained *in total* as a result of the impact of the project. A point raised by Richard Price is relevant here. Unless we *look* for outcomes, we won't know that they exist. And worse - we will carry on our mental health promotion as if they don't exist. So unless we look beyond the impact of interventions and policy towards the wider and longer term outcomes, we will never generate a sufficiently compelling empirical evidence base for our work. (Price 1997)

So links between impact and outcome need to be made to include such things as listed in table 3 below. In short, all of these points are indicators of the likely *allocative efficiency* of an intervention. Clearly, focusing on indicators of this sort would prevent resources being wasted on interventions which even if expertly and enthusiastically managed and well funded are never, in principle, going to produce anything other than short term, unsustainable, isolated results. The list could be argued as constituting the sort of checklist that commissioners or those responsible for Health Improvement Plans would (or at least should) be interested in, rather than the more 'project-management' sort of checklist (which concern technical efficiency only) which are the ones usually seen. These technical, operational issues are well within the bounds of good mental health promotion specialists to construct for themselves.

Effectiveness of Pipe-end Technology in Mental Health Promotion

Having identified some of the questions that could or should be asked about how the impact of an mental health promotion intervention or policy contrib-

Table 3: Linking impact to outcome - some basic questions

Supportive research	What empirical backing is already available about impact and outcomes for the intervention, and how translatable is this from researched to the operational situation?
Underpinning theory	What level of support is there from the available theory that an intervention will contribute to the desired mental health gain?
Comprehensiveness	How comprehensively does the intervention acknowledge systemic relationships between micro, meso, and macro levels?
Complementarity	How complementary is the intervention in relation to other elements of mental health?
Cumulative Potential	How cumulative is the impact of the intervention likely to be throughout the future of the targeted individuals or communities?
Congruency	To what extent is the impact of the intervention in harmony with the impacts of other related interventions or policies?
Sustainability	For the target group involved in the intervention, how sustainable is the impact likely to be? How sustainable is this intervention given the available resources and the numbers to be targeted?
Timescale; 'Causality'	What can realistically be claimed over and above theimpact of the intervention in terms of the timescale before outcome changes are achieved? And is this timescale realistic or fanciful?
Confounding factors (Other Impacts)	What factors are likely to get in the way and thus diminish the effect of the intervention impact on its outcomes? This is to reiterate the point made about congruency.
Coverage	What proportion of the *whole* target population is covered by the immediate target group involved in the intervention? Is this acceptable? Or does the intervention simply perpetuate inequalities?
Penetration	How might the impact of the intervention on its immediate target group 'ripple out' into the wider target population? Is this acceptable? Or does the intervention simply perpetuate inequalities?
Overall Health Improvement	Taking all the above questions into account, what is the overall *allocative efficiency* of the intervention likely to be?

185

utes to mental health more generally, it is appropriate to look at the case of one specific example of mental health intervention, namely mental illness services. The recent emphasis on 'Evidence - Based Practice' quite rightly asks difficult questions of mental health promotion as it should also ask about mental illness services. As I have argued above, a move towards proactive allocative evaluation would serve to base our practice on much sounder theoretical as well as empirical research evidence but this applies just as much to mental illness services as it does to mental health promotion. Our response to a cal for evidence based practice in mental health promotion ought not to assume that evaluations currently applied to what might be called "pipe – end" mental health intervention constitutes a paradigm of good practice that we need to fall into line with. In other words, don't assume the evaluation playing field is level, because it isn't. By "pipe – end" mental health promotion, I am using an observation made by Harrision (1996). This concept originates in pollution control and other technologies that place all the resources to control pollution at the end of the pipe instead of looking more fundamentally at the production processes to cut down pollution at source. Another parallel is 'quality control' which acts 'at the pipe end' in rejecting below standard product, compared with 'quality assurance' which works to improve production processes so that mistakes don't occur in the first place. In many, many industries, it has been recognised that an urgent *reframing* of the problem was required in order to put in place a less wasteful, more efficient *systemic* solution. **This need for reframing is the challenge facing health care provision today.** For a wide range of preventable illness, and especially perhaps, mental health problems, we need to move our thinking and our strategies away from pipe-end technology, which waits for people to become ill, before we intervene. Pipe end technologies do not address the potentially large number of people waiting to be ill. This is clearly an important ethical point but there are other issue that need raising as well.

Firstly, in terms of conceptual rigour, the pipe-end professions exhibit conceptual confusions about the epistemological status of mental health and mental illness : a) by failing to adequately acknowledge the essentially subjective nature and social determinants of health and dis-ease, and b) by developing interventions based on this reductionist, context-less view of health. As Schofield eloquently puts it,

> The psychiatrist has expanded the domain of mental illness to include all degrees and kinds of psychological distress, failing to appreciate that the human suffers pain not because he is sick but because he is human. Schofield (1964).

This re-emphasises points about conceptual clarity made earlier in the paper. Secondly, the evaluation of mental illness intervention is not always convincing. A recent estimate is that the relapse/readmission rate in clinical psychiatry is 73%. (quoted by Harrison, 1996) This picture of ineffective interventions being promulgated on the back of poor evidence of effectiveness fits into a wider paucity of evidence in the NHS as a whole. For example, "Only 20% of Health Service interventions have been evaluated by double blind clinical trials" Riley (1995).

Finally, in order to compare like with like, evaluating the effectiveness of pipe-end interventions compared with more 'upstream' or systemic mental health promotion needs to be done at the input as well as the impact level. As an illustration, the total funding available for specialist health promotion work is on average £1.23 per head of population, (which is about 0.3% of a DHA budget) of which only £0.81 is described as 'core' funding. The range of expenditure is between £0.38 and £5.15. (French and Hilditch 1995) This has to be shared amongst all the health topic areas and settings. So clearly the budget for specialist mental health promotion work is very small. In comparison, when we look at the cost of pipe-end intervention we see that the 23% of an average health authority/health board budget spent on mental illness services is equivalent a spending *per head* of the population of between £30 and £40. Many more detailed comparisons of this kind are needed so that meaningful comparisons of pipe-end and systemic interventions can be made in mental health promotion.

Discussion

The paper has used the work of Labonte and Robertson to show that thinking about mental health promotion practice and evaluation is likely to fall within two distinct and competing paradigms. To an extent it would seem that the assumptions identified in each paradigm are contradictory and incommensurate – you either believe in one single reality or you don't; you either believe that the purpose of research is to search for a shared, negotiated meaning, or you don't. So an important point here is that these are fundamental issues and it would not makes sense to talk of 'choosing' between these positivist and the social constructionist tradition. We can choose between methodology (e.g. qualitative or quantitative), or between method (e.g. survey or case study), or instrument (e.g. questionnaire or focus group). And although qualitative methodology is often indicative of a social constructionist ontology, and a quantitative methodology indicative of a positivist one, this is not an inalienable connection. Thus, the fundamental differences are not between research in-

187

struments, methods or methodologies, but between the positivist and the social constructionist traditions or paradigms.

The implication of this analysis is that there seems to me to be no way that we can evaluate which tradition or paradigm is superior. The differences are about belief and assumption. The positivist would want to argue that their beliefs and assumptions are *true* whilst the social constructionist would want to argue that their beliefs and assumptions make more *sense* – either claim of course rests on the paradigm being defended. I would want to argue that in the case of mental health at least, the history of treating this positivistically has hardly been convincing in its effectiveness or defendable in its ethics whereas the more inclusive, holistic, systemic options offered within a social constructionist account do make more sense. But the main point here is that just because a mental health promotion intervention is evaluated within say, a positivist paradigm this sort of evaluation cannot be said to be in any way superior to a social constructionist evaluation. No one can or should claim that one is inherently better than the other – they are just different and each produces a different account of the intervention. It is simply not profitable or philosophically accurate to claim that for example, qualitative findings are inferior to the results of a quantitative survey – each give a different view of the reality being investigated.

Another point concerns the evaluation process. In terms of traditions and paradigms, then of course the positivist view may hold that only one sort of evaluation finding (e.g. the outcome) is relevant whereas the social constructionist would hold that evaluation at each stage of the research contributes valid and important (but different) aspect of the intervention. Further, whilst the positivist would be looking for *the* truth about the impact or outcome of the intervention, the social constructionist would be looking for the emergence of varying and competing truths. Another important difference concerns the timing of the evaluation process with positivist research focusing traditionally on the product of the intervention leaving evaluation therefore to the last. A more social constructionist view would hold that the evaluation process cannot be methodologically or ethically disentangled given that no evaluation can be value or impact free on the intervention being evaluated. This view would want evaluation to be in at the start and with this view of evaluation, it may well be possible to ask searching questions (as in fig 3) about a proposed intervention well before time and resources are committed to it. Bearing in mind the possibilities on this view of competing versions of 'what the intervention is for' (i.e. different theories of the problem), then questions can be asked about 'taken for granted' and possibly over-simplistic intentions such as 'improving mental health' or 'reducing stigma' or 'improving coping skills'.

Conclusions

This paper has argued that in evaluating or researching mental health promotion, one fundamental issue to be included is how an intervention is conceptualising 'mental health'. How various features or elements of mental health are operationalised in both the intervention and the research are also important. Further, just as thinking about mental health is likely to focus on one or other tradition or paradigm, so thinking about the evaluation of mental health promotion intervention will also be oriented within one paradigm or the other. Whilst it is possible to choose between methodologies, methods, and research instruments, it does not seem to me to be possible to choose between paradigms. There are fundamental differences between the positivist and the social constructionist traditions/paradigms and each have competing views about not only what mental health is but also how it can and should be promoted and how interventions can and should be evaluated. Although I feel strongly that the positivist tradition has not been very useful to the promotion of mental health, and that the assumptions and beliefs within the social constructionist paradigm seem to me make more *sense* of mental health promotion, I also want to acknowledge that there seems to me to be no way that we can evaluate which tradition or paradigm is superior. Each give a different view of the reality being investigated and make different claims about the status of their findings. Rather than try to *prove* the superiority of one paradigm or other I simply think it behoves all who work in mental health promotion as either practitioners or researchers to be *reflexive* about their practice, and acknowledge the paradigmatic origins and limitations of their assumptions and beliefs.

In terms of the implications of holding one paradigmatic view or the other, I have briefly identified some issues regarding the complexities of the evaluation process and argued that as far as mental health promotion is concerned, researchers coming from a social constructionist tradition will be looking for very different issues in their evaluation than positivist researchers. There would also be important differences in terms of the claimed status of the research findings, the process of the research, and in particular, how related the evaluation should be to the intervention itself. Important points here are the extent to which evaluation can and should begin before an intervention has started, and the sort of 'proof' or certainties that researchers think they can legitimately produce.

In mental health promotion, conceptual issues to do with its evaluation and research have not been widely addressed. Yet it seems clear that just as with the issue of mental health itself, considerable conceptual complexities occur within the research field and further debate in this area will no doubt be needed. The danger in not addressing the problems here is that as Labonte and Robertson have argued, good mental health promotion interventions will continue to be evaluated in inappropriate and unrealistic ways. If we are not clear at least about the limits of what can be expected from mental health promotion, we are bound to end up disappointed, disillusioned or both.

References

Adams, L. and Armstron, E. (1996) *From Analysis to Synthesis 2: the Revenge*. Unpublished workshop report.

Caplan, R. and Holland, R. (1990) 'Rethinking Health Education Theory', *Journal of Health Education*. 49(1) pp. 10-12.

Drucker, P. (1977) *Management*. Pan Books, London.

French, J. and Adams, L. (1986) ' From Analysis To Synthesis', *Health Education Journal* 45 (2).

French, J. and Hilditch, K. (1995) *Health promotion Unit Funding survey.* North Cumbria Health Development Unit.

Harrison, D. (1996) 'Health Gain and Health Promotion', *Paper presented to the 6th Health Promotion Managers' Conference,* October, 1996.

Health Education Authority (1997) *Quality Framework for Mental Health Promotion*, London, Health Education Authority.

Hosman, C. (1996) 'The Case for Functionally Related Fields', *Paper presented at the 6th European Conference on the Promotion of Mental Health*, September, 1996.

MacDonald, G. (1993) 'Defining the goals and raising the issues' in D. R. Trent & C. Reed (eds), *The Promotion of Mental Health* Vol.2, Ashgate, Aldershot.

MacDonald, G. (1994) *Promoting Mental Health?* Health Education Authority, London.

MacDonald, G. and O'Hara, K. (1996) *Position paper on mental health promotion.* Society of Health Education and Promotion Specialists.

McLeroy et al (1994) 'Social Science theory in health education: time for a new model?', *Health Education Journal* 1994, pp 305-312.

Price, R. (1997) Keynote Paper presented to the Ayrshire International Conference on Mental Health Promotion , April, 1997.

Riley (1995) *Releasing Resources to Achieve Health Gain*, Radcliffe Medical Press.

Schofield, W. (1964) *Psychotherapy: the purchase of friendship,* Prentice Hall, Englewood Cliffs, New Jersey.

Smee (1995) in *Releasing Resources to Achieve Health Gain,* Radcliffe Medical Press, London.

Trent, D. (1993) 'The concept of mental health' in *Promoting Mental Health: Everyone's Business,* N.W. Surrey Health Authority.

Tudor, K. (1992) 'Community Mental Health Promotion: a Paradigm Approach', in D. R. Trent (ed) *The Promotion of Mental Health Volume 1,* Ashgate, Aldershot.

Tudor, K. (1996) *Mental Health Promotion*, Routledge, London.

20 Mental Health Promotion: Theory and Practice Insights from a Literature Review

NATASHA MAUTHNER, MICHAEL KILLORAN-ROSS AND
JANE BROWN

Abstract

This article reports on a literature review of interventions specifically identified as emanating from a mental health promotion (as opposed to prevention) paradigm. A number of recurring debates within the field were identified, including: language and terminology; defining 'mental health'; models of mental health promotion; the use of over-generalised concepts; values, beliefs and assumptions implicit in mental health promotion interventions; diversity in what gets called mental health promotion and who does mental health promotion. The paper concludes by highlighting key issues critical to the future development of mental health promotion: the implications of mental health promotion being at an embryonic stage of development; the need for greater reflexivity; the need for integration; issues concerning the professional identity and practice in the mental health promotion field.

Introduction

Over the last decade, mental health promotion has become an increasingly important feature of health policy at local, national and international levels (e.g. CRAG, 1994; Department of Health, 1994, 1996; Lehtinen et al., 1997). The current incidence and prevalence of psychological ill-health, the limited financial and human resources available to provide treatment and rehabilitation services, and increasing demands by the public for care have necessitated strategic development of mental health promotion and prevention alternatives (Albee, 1959). Despite this political imperative, the emerging field of mental health promotion faces uncertainty and confusion over its identity, objectives and future. In particular, the lack of a coherent framework and the need for conceptual clarity have been identified as key issues, and considerable efforts have been made to develop models of mental health promotion (e.g. Trent, 1992; Tudor, 1996; MacDonald and O'Hara, 1998).

The confusion within the field of mental health promotion is not only of theoretical but also of practical concern since it affects our professional practice on a day to day basis. As researchers and practitioners in the field, we find that when conducting collaborative or multidisciplinary work much of our time is spent debating fundamental issues such as 'what is mental health' and 'what is mental health promotion'. For example, over the last 18 months, we have been writing a report on mental health promotion for young people in collaboration with a senior mental health promotion officer, a health promotion manager and a consultant in public health. The report is for the Scottish Needs Assessment Programme (SNAP) which was set up by the Scottish Forum for Public Health Medicine. SNAP aims to ensure that needs assessment makes a measurable impact on health outcomes by contributing to effective purchasing of health care. It also aims to raise awareness of health needs which the public or Health Boards may not have recognised, and provide evidence as to why they are important issues.

The rather tortuous process of putting together this report exemplifies for us many of the current difficulties with mental health promotion. Many of our discussions have revolved around how to define 'mental health' and 'mental health promotion'. How broad or narrow should our definition of mental health be? Should we include severe mental health problems, mild mental health problems, positive mental health or all of these? Should we use a model of mental health promotion, and if so, which one? Perhaps the most contentious issue is what examples of successful and 'effective' mental health promotion initiatives with young people should be included. The central problem is that this report is aiming to raise the profile of mental health *promotion* (not prevention) in young people. In order to do this we have to have some means of proving its effectiveness. However, we have found very few written reports of mental health *promotion* initiatives which have been evaluated and our literature review of effective interventions comprises principally prevention studies. We also struggle with contradictions between, on the one hand, our definition of mental health and our model of mental health promotion which emphasise individual, structural and socio-economic dimensions, and on the other hand, our review of 'effective' mental health promotion interventions which comprises predominantly individualistic, psychological in-

192

terventions focusing on coping skills or cognitive processes. As a result of these tensions and contradictions, our report is somewhat disjointed. While it advocates the importance of mental health promotion in addition the prevention and treatment of mental 'disorders', it fails to provide any kind of evidence that mental health promotion works.

We use this SNAP report as a way of illustrating the conceptual and theoretical problems which plague the field of mental health promotion, and which affect our daily practice in a very real way. This SNAP report, and the tensions and discussions surrounding it, also provided the impetus for the piece of work which we report on here. In an effort to reach greater clarity concerning the current state of the field of mental health promotion we decided to conduct a critical literature review of interventions specifically identified as emanating from a mental health promotion paradigm. While existing so-called mental health promotion effectiveness reviews claim to reflect both prevention and promotion paradigms, they generally neglect work carried out within the latter (e.g. Hosman and Veltman, 1994; Hodgson et al., 1996; NHS Centre for Reviews and Dissemination, 1997; Tilford et al., 1997). They include largely randomised controlled trials published in peer-review journals and derived from a prevention paradigm. These reviews exclude explicit mental health promotion initiatives which are rarely published in mainstream academic outlets. Indeed, as this review found, mental health promotion interventions, where they are documented at all, are more likely to be reported in the 'grey literature' including newsletters, conference proceedings, briefing papers and reports.

Aims

Our aim in conducting this literature review was not simply to review and categorise existing mental health promotion interventions. Rather, the review process was a means of critically reflecting on the field of mental health promotion and identifying key areas of debate, as well as reflecting on the way forward for the field. The overall aim was to review past and current literature specifically identified as emanating from a mental health promotion paradigm. Specific objectives included: an analysis of the theoretical definitions and models of mental health promotion; a review of the broad range of mental health promotion activities; and an examination of the extent to which mental health promotion principles are implemented in practice both in the context of specific initiatives and more broadly within the field.

Methods

Four strategies were used in conducting our literature review. First, in order to establish the scope and extent of activities defined as mental health promotion, we examined the published conference proceedings from the series of European mental health promotion conferences (Trent and Reed, 1992, 1993, 1994, 1995, 1996, 1997). This initial strategy was important since this source was to provide the most extensive documentation of mental health promotion initiatives. Second, we searched databases including the Health Education Board for Scotland's own database (1989-1998) with the aim of locating relevant literature both in Britain and internationally. Third, we used key documents and texts (e.g. Clifford Beers Foundation, 1996; Health Education Authority, 1997; Health Education Board for Scotland, 1998; Hosman & Veltman, 1994; MacDonald & O'Hara, 1998; Tilford et al., 1997; Tudor, 1996). Finally, key commentators and agencies (e.g. Health Education Authority; Health Education Board for Scotland; Health Promotion Wales) in the field of mental health promotion were contacted and their opinions solicited on the sources used in this review and recommendations for further reading. This strategy proved very useful. As well as providing us with some of the grey literature, and some texts which we had not located, these key individuals had considerable knowledge and information themselves which is not documented elsewhere.

Main Findings

Our literature review identified a number of recurring debates and problems within the field of mental health promotion.

Language and Terminology

There has been much discussion of what language to use when talking about emotional, psychological and mental health and well being. There has been a move away from using the term 'mental illness' to using the term 'mental health'. This move is partly an attempt to reduce the stigma attached to the notion of mental illness, and partly an indication that mental health services contain practices derived from beyond the confines of an illness model (Rogers and Pilgrim, 1997). However, the term mental health is still used by many to

194

talk about 'mental illness'; and in this sense mental health becomes redefined as pathology (Henden, 1992). This has lead many to suggest that this change in language is simply a politically correct move with no real shift in thinking (Rogers and Pilgrim, 1997). In an attempt to make this conceptual shift the term 'positive mental health' (e.g. Money, 1996) is increasingly being used although, as many point out, it is unclear exactly what this term means (Rogers and Pilgrim, 1997).

Defining 'Mental Health'

The issue of language and terminology is in turn related to debates regarding the concept of mental health and how to define it. Probably the most enduring and contentious debate has been mobilised around defining mental health (Tudor, 1996; Trent, 1995) and whether it is realistic to attempt to do so (see MacDonald, 1993). Many argue that greater clarity of definition is necessary for genuine and effective mental promotion (e.g. Braidwood, 1997; Evans, 1992; Trent, 1995; Money, 1996) and that the current lack of consensus is deeply problematic (Herron, 1997). How can we design interventions if we cannot define mental health? How can we move forward in the field of mental health promotion if we cannot reach a consensus on what exactly mental health is? Trent (1993 p561), for example, observes that: "The primary difficulty in promoting mental health is due in no small part to the lack of any reasonable definition of what mental health is, within the professionals and the general public at large". Trent (1995) takes an extreme stance maintaining that until the question of definition is clarified it is difficult to establish what actually constitutes a mental health promotion intervention or strategy. Others advocate pluralism and support the coexistence of a multiplicity of definitions which are seen as reflecting not so much an unresolved conceptual problem but rather the expression of different perspectives on mental health, each with its own benefits and limitations (Clifford Beers Foundation, 1996; Tudor, 1996; Health Education Board for Scotland, 1998). Another constituency of commentators suggest that it is simply not appropriate to define mental health. MacDonald and O'Hara (1998), for example, adopt a 'constructionist' position which recognises the significance of social context and the cultural specificity of any definition of mental health. They argue that there are ethical, philosophical and pragmatic reasons for not searching for a single definition of mental health (see also Herron and Springett, 1995).

Another area of debate and confusion concerns the definition of mental health promotion. Mental health promotion is a contested concept and commentators have noted that while there are clear ideas about what mental health promotion is *not* - namely, an illness centred, medicalised approach to mental health problems - there is less clarity as to what it *is* (Trent, 1993). Perhaps the most well rehearsed debate here is whether mental health promotion concerns the promotion of positive mental health, the prevention of mental health problems (e.g. Price, 1997; Hosman, 1997), or both of these. Another source of confusion is the gap between what mental health promotion is in theory and what it is in practice - this is particularly the case in relation to mental health promotion's aim to address structural issues and inequalities when in practice it focuses on the individual, or at most on the home, school or immediate community. Another problem is the fact that many of the studies we examined gave no explicit definition or model of mental health promotion although implicitly some kind of model or framework did inform the work that was being reported. Where definitions and models of mental health promotion are offered they do not appear to share a common conceptual base. For example, we found that the frameworks being used varied from developmental psychology (Hodgson et al., 1996), to psychoanalytic approaches (e.g. Jebali, 1993), to evolutionary and ethological approaches (e.g. Gilbert, 1992). Thus, mental health promotion draws on different disciplines and theoretical traditions and lacks a coherent theoretical base. Recently, however, some degree of consensus has emerged with MacDonald and O'Hara's (1998) model of mental health promotion being increasingly adopted by, for example, the Society of Health Education and Health Promotion Specialists (MacDonald and O'Hara, 1998), the Health Education Authority (Health Education Authority, 1997), and the Health Education Board for Scotland (Health Education Board for Scotland, 1998).

The Use of Over-generalised Concepts

A further problem we identified in our literature review is the use of over-generalised concepts which tends to characterise discussions of mental health promotion. Concepts such as 'empowerment', 'stress', 'self esteem,' 'coping skills', 'social support' and 'lay perspectives' are used without adequately defining them and as if they are unproblematic categories. There is an over reliance of these broad and homogenous concepts, with little attempts being made to clarify their meaning in particular in the contexts in which they are applied.

*Values, Beliefs and Assumptions Implicit in Mental Health Promotion
Interventions*

In conducting this literature review, we found that certain key values, beliefs
and assumptions remain implicit in accounts of mental health promotion interventions. In particular, specific value-laden views are put forward about
what it is to be human, what it is to be healthy, and what kind of society we
should live in. One example is the implicit view of 'human nature'. Humans
are constructed as relentlessly social since 'being social', being a member of
a supportive social network and a caring community are seen as critical to
mental health. This underpins much of what is described as mental health
promotion because the strengthening of social relationships and ties, especially familial relationships (e.g. Harrison, 1993), is represented as a key element of mental health promotion. 'Being social' and having strong and
supportive social networks are assumed to bring benefits, and the possible
negative impact of social support on mental health is rarely addressed.

*Diversity in What Gets Called Mental Health Promotion and Who Does
Mental Health Promotion*

We also found that there was striking diversity in mental health promotion
practice. A very broad range of activities are described and reported as 'mental health promotion', including: parenting and child focused initiatives; work
place based schemes that tend to deal with stress; life crisis based interventions including bereavement counselling; anger management; psychological
well being and gay identity; exercise and mental health; support for individuals in the event of disasters; and laughter clinics. Furthermore, there is also a
very wide range of allied professions who 'do' mental health promotion in
addition to mental health promotion specialists, including community psychiatric nurses, health visitors and general practitioners. The term mental
health promotion is used so widely and broadly by so many different professional groups that it becomes difficult to define and draw clear boundaries
around mental health promotion and what exactly it is.

197

Taking Mental Health Promotion Forward

As a result of this literature we have identified a number of issues which we suggest are important for the development and future of mental health promotion and for taking the field forward.

Mental Health Promotion is at an Embryonic Stage of Development

The first point seems an obvious one and that is that mental health promotion is at an early stage of development. Although many of the ideas and ideals underpinning mental health promotion can be traced back to the Mental Hygiene Movement of the early 1900s and to key figures such as Clifford Beers, mental health promotion as we know it today first emerged in the 1980s. The early stage of development of mental health promotion is an important consideration when assessing the stage of debate in the field - for example in relation to the issues of language, definitions of mental health, and models of mental health promotion. From this perspective, the recurrence of these debates and controversies is not so much a problem or limitation within the field, as a necessary stage in the development of mental health promotion.

The Need for Greater Reflexivity in the Field of Mental Health Promotion

The second point which has emerged from our literature review is that the field of mental health promotion in general, and those engaged in mental health promotion activities specifically, need to more reflexive. For example, we need to reflect on the historical emergence of mental health promotion at this moment in time, and ask why there is so much interest in and concern with well being, quality of life, and positive mental health. We also need to analyse the political and economic context of this emergence and interest, and reflect on the historical genesis of mental health promotion as a movement, profession and practice. Here sociological approaches to understanding the emergence of specific social problems may have something to offer mental health promotion and illuminate why this interest in positive mental health and psychological well being have emerged at this particular time.

Mental health promotion is not just a theory or field of research, policy and practice. It is also a political reform movement advocating a shift of priorities, resources and power in alignment with a broader way of thinking about mental health and well being (see also Seedhouse, 1998; Signal, 1998).

198

We need to consider how the political and ideological basis of mental health promotion sits side by side with its quest for scientific status and legitimacy.

Similarly, we have discussed how certain beliefs, values and assumptions are implicit within mental health promotion interventions, in particular that mental health promotion is a pro-social activity because the strengthening of social ties and family relationships are integral to mental health promotion. Those engaged in mental health promotion need to be more reflexive about these as well as other values which they may inadvertently be imposing on others.

The Need for Integration in the Field of Mental Health Promotion

Although mental health promotion theory draws on a number of feeder disciplines including sociology, psychology, epidemiology and education when we reviewed accounts of mental health promotion activities we found that in practice mental health promotion appears as an isolated enclave remote and detached from mainstream debates and developments in the social sciences. One example is mental health promotion's attempts to address both individual and structural issues. Theoretical discussions about agency and structure are well rehearsed within the social sciences and mental health promotion could usefully draw upon these (e.g. Giddens, 1984). Another example is work on lay perspectives of mental health and the failure to theorise the status of these lay perspectives. In particular, lay perspectives are taken at face value and generally few references are made to the social science methodology literature which critically addresses the status of accounts as 'versions of reality' (e.g. Olesen, 1994).

Professional Identity and Practice in the Mental Health Promotion Field

One of the key questions to emerge from our literature review concerns the core identity of mental health promotion and what it is that is unique about it. What does mental health promotion offer that is not provided elsewhere by other professional groups? The scope of its activities is so broad and extensive that, inevitably, its potential to overlap with the remit of other professional groups is enormous (Health Education Authority, 1997). Perhaps it is particularly difficult to establish a professional niche when the niche could be found in so many different places. Consequently, this raises questions regarding the boundaries of mental health promotion and the ways in which the role of mental health promotion specialists differs and converges with the remit of allied professions, including psychology, health promotion and health education. This issue concerning the core identity of mental health promotion is critical to its future particularly in the context of economic constraints within the National Health Service and negative perceptions of mental health promotion among, for example, general practitioners (e.g. Maw, 1996).

We suggest that in order to begin to clarify some of these issues an empirical study of professional practice in mental health promotion in the United Kingdom would be worthwhile including interviews with mental health promotion specialists, health promotion managers and commissioners and members of allied professions such as psychiatrists, and psychologists. Here, we suggest a number of issues which could usefully be explored within an empirical study.

An urgent first task is to map the extent and scope of current activity in the United Kingdom as we found that systematic documentation of the extent of current mental health promotion activities remains rather limited and uncoordinated. Furthermore, research findings from other cultural locations, most notably from North America, are imported, used as an evidence base and assumed to be directly relevant to the British context. It would be more helpful to map and collate information about home grown interventions. Some of the questions we still need answers to and which might clarify the way forward for mental health promotion are: What range of activities are currently defined as mental health promotion? What range of professionals provide mental health promotion? What are the constraints on mental health promotion practice and on the implementation of mental health promotion theory? How do mental health promotion specialists experience and view their professional role? To what extent do they effectively work in a multidisciplinary way, alongside for example, psychology, psychiatry, nursing and social work? What model of mental health promotion do mental health promotion specialists work with? To what extent can these theoretical models be translated into the development of services and interventions; and what are the constraints on this process? Where should mental health promotion specialists be located e.g. within or outwith the National Health Service? What training is provided for mental health promotion practitioners, and what are their training needs? How do mental health promotion specialists see the future of mental health promotion? How is mental health promotion perceived by the allied professions? Can an economic or scientific case be made for mental health promotion?

An empirical investigation of these and other issues would have practical uses both in terms of strategic planning and training at the in-service level.

Summary and Conclusions

Mental health promotion is in a period of transition in Great Britain. Echoing the development of other professions in moving from the market place with apprenticeship training to the University with professional schools, there are now designated mental health promotion officers with specific remits in mental health promotion in most, if not all, health promotion departments throughout the United Kingdom. This welcome change is associated with a range of developmental difficulties which have been explored within this paper. Recurring debates and problems within the field cohere around issues in language and terminology, in definitions of mental health, in models of mental health promotion and in associated issues such as the use of over-generalised concepts and the implicit value base on which practice has been developed. Further research within the area is required if the potential of the field is to be realised.

References

Albee, G. W. (1959) *Mental Health Manpower Trends*, Basic Books, New York.

Braidwood, E. (1997) 'In search of a shared concept?', in D. R. Trent, & C. A. Reed, (eds), *Promotion of Mental Health, Volume 6*, Avebury, Aldershot.

Clifford Beers Foundation. (1996) *Enhanced Mental Health Promotion and Prevention in Europe: A Policy Paper*, The Clifford Beers Foundation, Stafford.

CRAG Working Group on Mental Health (1994) *Primary Prevention in Mental Health*, Department of Health, Scottish Office Edinburgh.

Department of Health (1994) *Health of the Nation Key Areas Handbook: Mental Illness (Second Edition)*, HMSO, London.

Department of Health (1996) *On the State of the Public Health*, HMSO, London.

Evans, J. (1992) 'What is mental health and how can we promote it?', *Nursing Times*, 88, pp. 54-56.

Giddens, A. (1984) *The Constitution of Society*, Polity Press, Cambridge.

Gilbert, P. (1992) 'An evolutionary approach to the conceptualisation of mental health/theoretical issues', in Dennis R Trent, & C. Reed, (eds), *Promotion of Mental Health, Volume 1*, Avebury, Aldershot.

Harrison, M. (1993) 'Home-start: support, friendship and practical help for young families under stress', in D. R. Trent, & C. Reed, (eds), *Promotion of Mental Health, Volume 2*, Avebury, Aldershot.

Health Education Authority (1997) *Mental Health Promotion: A Quality Framework*, Health Education Authority, London.

Health Education Board for Scotland (1998) *Mental Health Promotion: A Strategic*

Statement, Health Education Board for Scotland Edinburgh.

Henden, J. (1992) 'The changing language of mental health/theoretical issues', in D. R. Trent, & C. Reed, (eds.), *Promotion of Mental Health, Volume 1*, Avebury, Aldershot.

Herron, S. & Springett, J. (1995) 'Mental health: the lay perspective', in D. R. Trent, & C. Reed, (eds), *Promotion of Mental Health, Volume 4*, Avebury, Aldershot.

Herron, S. (1997) 'The cloudy waters of mental health' in D. R. Trent, & C. Reed, (eds), *Promotion of Mental Health, Volume 6*, Ashgate, Aldershot.

Hodgson, R., Abbasi, T., & Clarkson, J. (1996) 'Effective mental health promotion: a literature review', *Health Education Journal*, 55, pp. 55-74.

Hosman, C. (1997) Developing promotion and prevention in mental health: a European perspective. Ayrshire International Mental Health Promotion Conference 1997, Troon, Scotland.

Hosman, C. M. H. and Veltman, N. E. (1994) *Prevention in Mental Health: Review of Effectiveness of Health Promotion and Health Education*, University of Nijmegen, Nijmegen, The Netherlands.

Jebali, C. (1993) 'The Implication of Using Women Centred Therapy in the Provision of Positive Mental Health Care', in D. R. Trent, & C. Reed, (eds), *Promotion of Mental Health, Volume 2*, Avebury, Aldershot.

Lehtinen, V., Riikonen, E., & Lahtinen, E. (1997) *Promotion of Mental Health on the European Agenda*, Stakes, Helsinki.

MacDonald, G. & O'Hara, K. (1998) *Ten Elements of Mental Health, its Promotion and Demotion: Implications for Practice*, Society of Health Education and Health Promotion Specialists.

MacDonald, G. (1993) 'Defining the goals and raising the issues in mental health promotion', in D. Trent, & C. Reed (eds), *Promotion of Mental Health, Volume 2*, Avebury, Aldershot.

Money, M. (1996) 'Mental health and mental illness: a positive community approach', *The Journal*, pp. 56-58.

NHS Centre for Reviews and Dissemination (1997) 'Mental health promotion in high risk groups', *Effective Health Care*, 3, pp. 1-12.

Olesen, V. (1994) 'Feminisms and models of qualitative research', in N. K. Denzin & Y. S. Lincoln (eds), *Handbook of Qualitative Research*, Sage, London.

Price, R. H. (1997) Progress on Promotion and Prevention in the United States. Ayrshire International Mental Health Promotion Conference 1997, Troon, Scotland.

Rogers, A., & Pilgrim, D. (1997) 'The contribution of lay knowledge to the understanding and promotion of mental health', *Journal of Mental Health*, 6(1), pp. 23-35.

Seedhouse, D. (1998) 'Mental health promotion: problems and possibilities', *International Journal of Mental Health Promotion*, 1, pp. 5-14.

Signal, L. (1998) 'The politics of health promotion: insights from political theory', *Health Promotion International*, 13, pp. 257-263.

Tilford, S., Delaney, F., & Vogels, M. (1997) *Review of the Effectiveness of Mental Health Promotion Interventions*, NHS Centre for Reviews and Dissemination and

Health Education Authority, England.

Trent, D. (1992) 'Breaking the Single Continuum', in D. R. Trent, & C. Reed (eds) *Promotion of Mental Health, Volume 1,* Avebury, Aldershot.

Trent, D. (1993) 'The promotion of mental health: fallacies of current thinking', in D. R. Trent, & C. Reed (eds), *Promotion of Mental Health, Volume 2,* Avebury, Aldershot.

Trent, D. (1995) 'You say prevention, I say promotion', in D. Trent, & C. Reed (Eds), *Promotion of Mental Health, Volume 4,* Avebury, Aldershot.

Trent, D., & Reed, C. (1992) *Promotion of Mental Health, Volume 1,* Avebury, Aldershot.

Trent, D., & Reed, C. (1993) *Promotion of Mental Health, Volume 2,* Avebury, Aldershot.

Trent, D., & Reed, C. (1994) *Promotion of Mental Health, Volume 3,* Avebury, Aldershot.

Trent, D., & Reed, C. (1995) *Promotion of Mental Health, Volume 4,* Avebury, Aldershot.

Trent, D., & Reed, C. (1996) *Promotion of Mental Health, Volume 5,* Avebury, Aldershot.

Trent, D., & Reed, C. (1997) *Promotion of Mental Health, Volume 6,* Avebury, Aldershot.

Tudor, K. (1996) *Mental Health Promotion: Paradigms and Practice,* Routledge, London.

Acknowledgements

The literature review on which this paper is based was funded by Community Health Care (NHS) Trust, Ayrshire and Arran. The Research Unit in Health and Behavioural Change is funded by the Chief Scientist Office of the Scottish Office Department of Health and the Health Education Board for Scotland. The views expressed in this communication are those of the authors not the funding bodies.

21 The Odin European Research on Preventing Depression: A Different Perspective

CLAIRE HAYES, CHRISTINE MURPHY AND THE ODIN GROUP

Abstract

Over the past two years Ireland, Finland, Norway, Spain, and UK, have been involved in jointly researching a psycho-educational approach to treating/preventing depression (The Odin research project), using an adaptation of Munoz's "Coping with Depression" Course as the group treatment (Munoz and Ying, 1993). Statistical analysis of the extensive data collected is currently being carried out, and the Partners** will present the results shortly. As the two instructors involved in giving the group treatment programmes in Ireland and the U.K. we would like to look at the research, not statistically, but from a different perspective – our own, and from that of some of the participants. We were struck by the many positive effects that we perceived in the participants during the course of the treatment programmes. A welcome and unexpected bonus was that similar positive effects were also evident in our own lives, thus convincing us further of the value of this work. Now that the treatment stage of the research is at a close we would like to share our experiences of running the groups with others, looking in a critical way at the benefits and restrictions of following a manualised prevention programme.

Odin in Context

"Odin" is the chosen mnemonic for "The Outcomes of Depression International Network", a European, multi-centre research group set up in 1996 to

205

provide data on the prevalence, risk factors and outcomes of depressive disorders in urban and rural areas within the European Union and to assess the impact of two psychological interventions on the outcome of depression and on health service and utilisation and costs (Dowrick et al 1998). The five participating centres are the UK, Ireland, Norway, Finland and Spain, with the first four countries studying the effects of a group psychoeducational intervention. This treatment followed the educational model described by Lewinsohn et al (1986) and Munoz and Ying (1993) with some modification so as to increase the content devoted to social support. The UK also used the individual intervention (Hawton and Kirk 1989), while Spain focused solely on the individual with no group intervention.

As the two therapists involved in running the intervention groups in Ireland and the UK, we were not involved in either the selection of the subjects or the evaluation of the treatment. However, we both were struck by the rapid changes that we perceived in the participants, as well as noticeable positive changes in our own personal lives. While the statistical analysis is currently being carried out, and the formal results will be presented by the Partners at a later date, we were interested in looking at what the participants remembered about the programme some months later, whether they had found it helpful or not, and what comments they had about the programme. Consequently we designed a brief open-ended questionnaire and sent it to all the participants. The replies are discussed below, followed by our own observations, but first we give a description of the group treatment, along with the rationale for using it in this research.

A Description of the Group Treatment Programme

The "Coping with Depression" course is a structured psycho-educational treatment developed by Lewinsohn and his associates (Lewinsohn, Antonucci, Breckenridge & Teri, 1984). The course is based on social learning theory (Bandura 1977), and sees depression as being associated with a decrease in pleasant activities and an increase in unpleasant activities (Lewinsohn et al 1986). The problems shown by individuals with depression are viewed as being due to behavioral and thinking patterns that can be unlearned or relearned. A cognitive-behavioural approach (Beck et al 1979, Ellis and Harper, 1961) is used in helping participants identify and challenge their thoughts, while at the same time increasing the number of pleasant activities they have on a daily basis. For the purpose of Odin an amended form of the "Coping with Depression" course by Munoz and Ying (1993) was piloted by therapists in U.K, Ireland, Norway and Finland during 1996. Following a review meeting early in 1997, it was decided that the order of some of the sessions would be changed and there would be some minor omissions with a greater emphasis placed on social support. This programme was then "taught" to participants over an eight-week period, with each "class" lasting 150 minutes (inclusive of a 30-minute tea break to encourage social support amongst participants). It was emphasised throughout that the programme was a "course" as opposed to therapy, and that participants would be expected to carry out regular homework assignments. It is called a course because it is explicitly used to teach people techniques to cope with the problems that are assumed to be related to their depression (Lewinsohn, Hoberman and Clarke 1989). In line with this the group leaders are seen more as instructors than therapists, and the participants are students, rather than patients (Cuijpers, 1998).

In the Irish and the UK sections of the Odin group intervention each class had three to eight members. Prior to the first session the participant's permission was necessary to inform their doctor/therapist of their attendance on the course and to enable video taping of the second session (for reliability purposes). Actively suicidal people, and/or those abusing drugs and alcohol were excluded. Handouts were given at each session to review core ideas and as preparation for classes. Each class started with an outline of material to be covered followed by a brief relaxation exercise. The course consisted of an introductory session looking at the purpose of the course, symptoms of depression and an explanation of the social learning theory. Subsequent modules focused on relaxation, social skills, cognitive skills and ways of increasing pleasant activities. While the course followed the set manual, it was agreed that each therapist would have flexibility as to the exact way she introduced the core ideas.

The rationale for such an intervention was based on much previous research highlighting that:

- Depression is a very common condition leading to disability and much socio-economic costs. Katon (1987) found that depression may be the most common medical or psychiatric disorder seen in medical care settings, occurring in up to 30% of patients seen by primary care physicians.
- Depression has an impact on the community greater than that of many chronic diseases (Croft-Jeffreys and Wilkinson1989, Ormel et al 1994).
- Depression in medical patients is largely overlooked or ignored by medical staff (Organista, Munoz and Gonzalez, 1994).
- Relapse is common, occurring in up to 75% of cases within 10 years (Thornicroft and Sartorius, 1993).

207

- Prevention of onset is particularly important because so many people are affected by it (Munoz, 1997).
- Research is needed to develop methods to prevent depression (Munoz et al. 1995).
- Cognitive-behavioural interventions are as effective as anti-depressant medication (Lewinsohn et al, 1989).
- Experience suggests that a number of persons who are typically resistant to psychotherapy are more amenable to an educational format in which they learn coping skills (Lewinsohn et al, 1989).
- As a group intervention the psychoeducational approach is more cost effective (Lewinsohn, 1989).
- The psycho-educational nature makes the course less stigmatizing than traditional therapy (Cuijper, 1998).
- The course has been found to have great potential as a preventative intervention for various groups of people at risk from depressive disorders (Lewinsohn et al, 1989).
- One of the most promising areas in which this intervention can be used is the prevention of depression, early case-finding and early treatment (Cuijper, 1998).

We need to improve our knowledge of the extent of depression in rural areas and to gain information on help seeking strategies and availability of health care (Dowrick et al 1998). Format of Groups:

	Offered	Attended all	Attended some	Did not attend
Ireland Urban 1	9	4	3	2
Ireland Urban 2	9	5	2	2
Ireland Rural 1	8	3	1	4
UK Urban	15	3	1	11
UK Pilot 1	8	3	1	4

Participants' Own Experiences of the Treatment Several Months After Completing It

The questionnaire we sent to all of the participants asked if (and when) they had completed the course, what they had remembered from it, the ideas they had found useful and whether the course had changed their view of the future in anyway. It also checked if they thought the number of sessions were adequate and asked for their comments on the homework exercises. Finally we

208

asked if they had kept in contact with any other members of the group, and if there was anything else they thought might be helpful for us to know. 50% of the people returned their questionnaires.

The following is a thematic representation of people's comments:

1. What Did People Remember From the Course?

- Supportive gathering - pleasant, warm, comforting.
- Shared experience *"being able to see other depressed people means I'm not so mental after all!"*
- Being in contact with other people stops the social isolation of depression.
- Positive thinking.
- Establishing routine relaxation.
- Dealing with the many facets of depression.
- Facing up to being in need of help.
- That prevention is better than cure.

2. What Ideas Covered During the Course Did You Find Helpful?

- Having more contact with positive people.
- Increasing pleasant activities.
- Controlling moods and feelings: *"to be successful you have to want to change your thoughts.", "I shout (silently!) at myself to stop."*
- Feeling in control: *It's me who has control of any changes I want to make."*
- Monitoring thoughts: *"Learning to change my thoughts."*
- Planning: *"I take my mind off sad thoughts by planning something to do.", "I keep a diary of things to do."*
- Small steps to change: *"One simple thing in your daily routine can relieve the tension.", "Changing just one thing is enough to start the ball rolling."*
- Stopping negative thinking: *"Catch yourself worrying.", "Changing just one thing is enough to start the ball rolling."*
- Using positive thinking: *" Make the most of what you have."*
- Breathing and relaxation techniques: *"knowing how to relax more."*
- Boosting self-esteem: *"I'm no worse than anyone else and I have a lot of good points.", "I respect myself more and tell myself I'm worth it!",*

"Taking time out for myself."
- Objectivity: *"I can view situations more objectively."*
- Awareness: *"I am beginning to reflect more."*
- Assertiveness: *"Now I'm not afraid to say "no" in a particular situation."*
- Keep calm!
- People remembered phrases used on the course - they said it reinforced things they already knew.

3. Did You Think 8 Sessions Were Enough?

Although we gained some informative qualitative information from the response that we got, as only 50% of group members responded to our questionnaire, the answers given to this question may not be truly representative of the groups as a whole.

Of the responders, *25%* said there were *just enough* sessions;
   75% would have liked *more* sessions.
   25% asked for *follow-up* reinforcement sessions.

4. Has the Course Changed Your View of the Future in Any Way?

- Recognising trigger situations and preventing future episodes: *"Now I can get on top of a situation and work through it, whereas before I would have been seriously depressed."*
- Able to shorten the length of depressive episodes.
- Knowledge that you get better: *"I know once I go into one I will come out the other end and they don't last as long as they used to."*
- Ability to progress: *"I feel I can go on."*

5. How Did You Feel About Your Homework?

- *"Interesting, enjoyable, a good challenge!"*
- *"Hard work filling in the long form."*
- *"Time pressure made it difficult to fit it in."*
- *"Thought-provoking."*
- *"Consolidates things by writing them down."*
- *"Writing it down made me face up to things."*

- "Sharing it with other people is a big step."
- "It drew family members into the work."
- "It helped me to remember the lecture."

6. Have You Kept in Contact With Other Members of the Course?

Of the responders:

> 75% said they had not kept in contact, 25% had met socially since the course.

7. Is There Anything Else You Found Helpful?

- "I think anyone who has had depression should do a course like this - it is a life saver."
- "Perhaps a tape or booklet could be given to each participant?"
- "I think there should be a follow-up course to see how people have changed, if at all."
- "More people should know about the help there is for them."
- "Suggestion - a short list of the skills learned could be compiled into a Thought For The Day booklet."
- Confidentiality helped (it provided a confiding relationship which was lacking) "It seemed to be easier to air views about family matters and other things."
- Reduced use of medication in some cases "I've been able to some off my depressive tablets using positive thinking."
- Increased interest in alternative therapies. "I have attended a herb class." "Now I use St John's Wort for depression."

Instructors' Experiences of the Group Intervention

Christine Murphy (U.K.)

For me the course encompassed all the words of wisdom and many proverbs that had been impressed on me through my life from family, teachers, religious etc. It reinforced the home truths, and reminded me of the simple message that my feelings could be changed by becoming aware of and changing my thoughts and actions. It was a hopeful, positive and practical message to work through with the participants. I worked through the homework with the group and, as they were recognising areas of change for themselves, my first step was to highlight my need to be more organised. This led me to start to use a diary properly and to plan ahead. The saying "never put off till tomorrow what you can do today", was a guideline for me. An accumulation of things I needed to do was a source of worry for me. This led me to listing each day the tasks I needed to get out of the way to enable me to fit in enjoyable events. The course teaches methods of becoming aware of positive and negative thoughts and working on accentuating the positive.

These methods are still having an effect on my thinking and hopefully a knock on effect on my family. The course highlighted the importance of meeting my own needs, one of which was to resume physical activity. With planning I was able to attend 3 or 4 sessions a week at the gym, I started cycling at weekends with my husband. The positive input of the course encouraged me to accept challenges that I may well have found excuses for not doing. The essence for me was to be courageous, to face life positively and to know that although it is a constant battle I am in control of the way I feel and have practical methods to draw on when feeling low or overwhelmed by what life may have to throw at me. The course fostered a feeling of goodwill and a sharing of ideas amongst the class. As the instructor I often felt moved by the participants obvious hard work and great effort.

Claire Hayes (Ireland)

Having given the treatment programme four times I can safely say I learned as much, if not more than the participants. Initially, during the pilot programme I found the idea of a manualised approach to treatment rigid and restricting. I felt unsure as to if, when and how much I could deviate from the written word in the text and felt slightly guilty and uneasy if I brought in other examples to illustrate certain points. The huge discrepancy between one of the participants who had a long history of recurring, serious depression and the other two (at times reluctant) volunteers was marked. I learned however that the programme, by its respectful, accepting nature has much to offer, and I was relieved when the review meeting held shortly afterwards emphasised that the manual was there to help, not hinder us. So long as we covered the core ideas, it was acceptable that individuals' style would vary. Immediately that relaxed and freed me to get on with the work. Get on with – I honestly did not expect to enjoy it to the extent I did. During the long wet, dark, winter nights, the mild spring evenings, and the warm summer I was constantly amazed by people's energy and determination to attend, to learn, and to fight to gain control over their own emotions. When I first became involved with Odin I was familiar with the basic principles of cognitive-behavioural therapy and had used them in a number of clinical settings. I liked the common-sense approach and I felt I was convinced of its benefits. I was wrong. The people who participated in Odin challenged me to actively make changes in my own life. Gradually I found I was "doing" rather than "thinking". I was actively planning "pleasant activities" on a regular basis, I was becoming more assertive in suggesting and initiating, and quite honestly I was having much more fun. My family and friends noticed the change and a few even asked if they could attend the next course! Incorporating the preventative measures emphasised in the course into my every day life definitely improved its quality.

In addition to my own internal changes it was humbling and gratifying to see people change and become lighter in a relatively brief period of time. I am curious as to what the final statistics will show but I personally am in no doubt but that it was a worthwhile, valuable experience. Some years ago, when I was first introduced to the basic principles of cognitive behavioural therapy a question I kept wondering was "why must people wait until they have depression before they learn ways of coping with it?" That question is in my mind more often now, and in the face of increasing psychological distress, unhappiness and unease I believe that psycho-education, such as this programme, has much to offer.

Conclusion

So what have we learned? The people who returned our questionnaires were all positive about the programme, the majority felt the course of eight sessions was not enough and some suggested follow-up courses. We have not mentioned those who dropped out of the programme, nor have we referred to rural/urban differences, nor indeed cross-cultural differences. As we did not have a full response to our brief questionnaires we are careful not to make wide general statements. Clearly the course is not for everyone. Joining a group is difficult and the courage of those who attended even one session must not be over-looked. While no obvious differences emerged between the two urban sites in Ireland and the U.K., the rural people in Ireland did seem much more tentative about becoming involved. The extra emphasis on support proved to be very important in helping people build up trust and confidence in each other, although it is of note that none of the Irish and few of the

British who responded remained in contact.

Finally, as instructors, we would like to acknowledge how important the support we received from our colleagues in Odin was to us. We felt part of a team, a team motivated to helping people improve their quality of life. A team with energy, enthusiasm and good humour. Antonuccio, Danton and DeNelsky (1995) remind us of the tendency to underestimate the power and cost-effectiveness of a caring, confidential psychotherapeutic relationship in the treatment of depression. As professionals working in this area we must also not underestimate the power and cost-effectiveness of a caring, support-ive team!

* The Odin Group is composed of academic colleagues and researchers currently working with ODIN. At 1 August 1998 they include Trine Anstorp, Jose Luis Ayuso-Mateos, Kirsten Benum, Pim Cuijpers, Ioana Davies, Juan Francisco Diez Manrique, Ioana Davies, Graham Dunn, Rhiannon Edwards, Abdelaziz Elneihum, Mette Finne, Fiona Ford, Andrés Gómez del Barrio, Claire Hayes, Alfonso Higuera, Ann Horgan, Clemens Hosman, Tarja Koffert, Fiona Johnstone, Nicola Jones, Lourdes Lasa, Marja Lehtilä, Catherine McDonough, Erin Michalak, Christine Murphy, Anna Nevra, Teija Nummelin, Helen Page, Andrea Schmenger and Jon Strype.

** Partners:
- Chrisopher Dowrick, Prof. of Primary Medical Care, University of Liverpool, U.K.
- Jose Luis Vazquez-Barquero, Prof. of Psychiatry, Hospital Universitario "Marques de Valdecilla" Santander, Spain.
- Greg Wilkinson, Prof. of Liaison Psychiatry, University of Liverpool, U.K.
- Clare Wilkinson, Prof. of General Practice, University of Wales College of Medicine, Wrexham, Wales.
- Ville Lehtinen, Research Prof. Stakes mental health research group, Turku, Finland.
- Odd Steffen Dalgard, Institute of Community medicine, University of Oslo/National Institute of Public Health, Oslo, Norway.
- Patricia Casey, Prof. Adult Psychiatry, University College Dublin, Ireland.

References

Antonuccio, D., Danton, W. G., and DeNelsky, G.Y. (1995). Psychotherapy versus medication for depression: Challenging the conventional wisdom with data. *Professional Psychology; Research and Practice.* Vol. 26, no. 6, pp. 574-585.

Bandura, A. (1977). *Social learning theory.* Englewood Cliffs, N.J.: Prentice-Hall.

Beck, A.T., Rush, A. J., Shaw, B.F., and Emery, G. (1979). *Cognitive therapy of depression.* New York, Guilford Press.

Croft-Jeffreys, C. and Wilkinson, G. (1989) Estimated cost of neurotic disorder in UK general practice in 1985. *Psychological Medicine,* Vol. 19, pp. 549-558.

Cuijpers, P. (1998). Psychoeducation in the prevention of depression. In Press.

Dowrick, C., Casey, P., Dalgard, O., Hosman, C., Lehtinen, V., Vazquez-Barquero, Wilkinson, G., et al (1998). Outcomes of Depression International Network (ODIN) Background, methods and field trials. *British Journal of Psychiatry vol. 72,359-363.*

Ellis, A. and Harper, R.A. (1961). *A Guide to Rational Living.* Hollywood, CA., Wilshire Books.

Katon, W. (1987). The epidemiology of depression In medical care. *International Journal In Medicine.* Vol. 17, pp. 93-112.

Lewinsohn, P.M., Antonucci, D.O., Breckenridge, J.S. and Teri, L. (1984) The coping with Depression Course. Eugene: Castilia Publishing Company.

Lewinsohn, P.M., Hoberman, H.M. and Clarke, G.N. (1989). The coping with depression course; Review and future directions. *Canadian Journal Behavioural Science.* Vol. 21, no. 4, pp. 470-493.

Lewinsohn, P. M., Munoz, R.F., Youngren, M. A., et al (1986) *Control your Depression.* New York: Prentice Hall.

Munoz, R.F. (1997). Preventing depression: A reality management approach. Paper presented as part of a symposium Applying Clinical Psychological Science to Prevention Trials for Unipolar Depression at the 105th Annual Convention of the American Psychological Association, August15-19.

Munoz, R.F., Ying, Y., Bernal, G., Perez-Stable, E., Sorenson, J., Hargreaves, W., Miranda, J. and Miller, L. (1995). Prevention of depression with primary care patients: A randomised controlled trial. *American Journal of Community Psychology,* vol. 23, no. 2, pp. 199-222.

Munoz, R.F. and Ying, Y. (1993) *The Prevention of Depression: Research and Practice.* Baltimore, MD: Johns Hopkins University Press.

Organista, K.C., Munoz, R.C. and Gonzalez, G. (1994). Cognitive-behavioural therapy for depression in low-income and minority medical outpatients: Description of a program and exploratory analyses. *Cognitive Therapy and Research,* vol. 18, no.3, pp. 241-259.

Ormel, J.,Koetter, M.W. and van Brink, W (1989) Measuring change with the General Health Questionnaire. Social Psychiatry and Psychiatric Epidemiology, 24.227-232.

Thornicroft, G. and Sartorius, N.(1993) The course and outcome of depression in different cultures: 10 year follow up of the WHO collaborative study on the assessment of depressive disorders. *Psychological Medicine,* Vol. 23, pp. 1023-1032.

22 Selling Mental Health Promotion

MICHAEL C. MURRAY

Introduction

All organizations perform two basic functions. They produce a good, a service, or an idea and they market it. This is true of all firms - from international giants such as Mazda to an exclusive French boutique. It is true of both profit-seeking firms and non-profit organizations (Boone & Kurtz -1992).

Health promotion departments are included!

The essence of this paper is to argue that unless we are able to effectively market our promotion/prevention strategies we will be failing to carry out an essential part of our role; the programme/strategy will not realise its full potential.

This paper will address the following issues in supporting a market orientated approach to "Selling Mental Health Promotion".

a) the empowering of programme participants;
b) the validity of continuing to utilise a product orientated approach in the design and implementation of mental health promotion/prevention strategies;
c) the need for health promoters to recognise that they are working within a changing environment and as such must confront a number of variables that are present within an emerging market economy;

d) the ability to identify and recognise the needs and wants of the different stakeholders involved in the programme;

e) the development of a balanced set of objectives with a balanced set of stakeholders.

Finally the paper will discuss a model that can be utilised to assist and encourage the different stakeholders to work creatively together in a collaborative approach and thereby help increase the effectiveness of the mental health promotion programme.

Empowerment

A fundamental attribute of health promotion is empowerment As *MacDonald (1997)* succinctly put it:

> *Health promotion involves empowerment, a process whereby individual people are encouraged to assert their own autonomy and esteem sufficiently to be able to identify their own agendas, rather than being told what to do or what is good for their health.*

Empowerment as we know relates to the giving of power and the authorising and enabling of others to play a part in the event.

We can illustrate this point by a very simple example. A mother wants her reticent small son, who incidentally dreams of being a footballer, to eat his vegetables. She could compel him to do as he was told at every meal and suffer the consequent problems. Alternatively she could explain how by eating the vegetables he will grow up stronger and healthier and hence a better footballer. The second, empowering approach, provides a reward system for both mother and son together with a more likely successful outcome.

Furthermore this simple example illustrates how effective programme implementation depends upon the recognition that all the parties (stakeholders) involved in the project need to have their needs met.They require a pay-off, whether this be in financial, health gain, self esteem or other terms.

Organisational Commitment

However, empowerment alone is not sufficient to ensure the success of the health promotion project. There is the need for a substantial degree of commitment from all stakeholders in the project.

In learning from the ideas of *Morgan (1997)* we note that the success of an organisation hinges upon the creation of shared meaning and shared understanding, because there have to be common reference points if people are to share and align their activities in an organised way.

As an organization is a group of people who are bonded together to achieve a common purpose *Schermerhorn et al (1997)*. Thus in the development and implementation of an effective promotion/prevention strategy we must build an effective team or organisation of people who understand and are committed to the aims and objectives of the project.

In *Simnett (1997)* the need for co-operation or partnership approach is also emphasised:

> *Many of the activities we need to invest in for health gain through health promotion work can only be delivered through partnerships between organisations, and between organisations and communities, to make a significant contribution to the achievement of health gain for local populations. This is done by building effective partnerships...*

Within industry or commerce this 'partnership' approach is perhaps a more straightforward proposition as the profit motive is the often over-riding common thread to hold the different stakeholders together.

A Product Orientated Approach

However in the past the issue of service delivery. In the NHS as a whole and to a significant degree in health promotion was perhaps much simpler with the need for a partnership approach not recognised or accepted. In reality a product/orientated approach *(Doyle 1997)* has been taken As *Kotler (1988)* puts it, the idea is that the organisation delivers products that it thinks will be good for the customer (patient). With high-tech medicine the view that developing technological supervisor treatments is the route to success is paramount. Hence clinicians make the decisions and little or no effort is made to encourage participation by patients and families. A hierarchical approach is adhered to and the patient is a recipient of the prescribed service.

But if health promoters accept the need for an empowerment and self-assertion they need to confront this philosophy and highlight concerns that can be attributed to this approach.

219

First of all who is to say the expert is right? *Seedhouse (1996),* puts forward the scenario that health promoters in the USA have been so successful in getting the anti-smoking message across that the USA public now perceive the risks from smoking to be much higher than they actually are. On the other hand, even after numerous anti-smoking campaigns increased numbers of women are smoking more. Furthermore we may not wish to take the view of the expert. To cut down on drinking may improve one's physical health but we may wish to continue to drink alcohol.

Perhaps, most importantly, to subscribe to such a top-down prescriptive policy not only serves to consolidate the medical model but also actively discriminates against the empowerment approach which is such a vital component in mental health promotion.

Consequently mental health promotion requires an approach which values the contribution that can be made by the individual and the different stakeholder groups within the boundaries set by a particular project.

A Market Orientated Approach

With the on-going governmental reforms, health promotion staff are now having to confront a multitude of changing variables in a workplace that is increasingly becoming a volatile market place. For example there is increasing regulation, decreasing outside funding, more aggressive competition for the limited funds, a variety of entrepreneurial posturing by health care providers and purchasers and of course the ascendancy of a more critical consumer population.

To be successful the health promoter has to market the product and not only to the traditional funder and recipient of the promotion project but to the different range of stakeholders whose input is essential for success e.g. staff, professional bodies, regulatory authorities etc.

Consequently the health promoter needs to learn the lessons from utilising the marketing concept which holds that the key to success consists in determining the needs and wants of the target markets and delivering the desired satisfactions more effectively and efficiently *Kotler (ibid).* The concept is simple. It is that the mental health promotion programme should be seen from the point of view of its final result from the recipient(s) point of view.

The Model: A Partnership Approach

So how can we develop a model or process to help ensure the efficient mental health promotion project is implemented in an effective manner and meets the need of those stakeholders integral to the success of the programme? Perhaps a first step is to recognise the long tradition of successful marketing in the commercial, profit-orientated world and in turn be prepared to heed lessons from that experience by utilising marketing and business strategy techniques. Marketing is about meeting the needs of the organisation's customers (clients) through offering and exchanging values with different stakeholders to gain their cooperation and thereby meet the organisation and stakeholder goals. It is as true of health promotion departments as it is of the commercial, for profit corporation. Strategy is the set of plans, decisions and objectives adopted to achieve the goals.

Thus the model set out below is proposed as an example as to how we can pursue this formula. For illustrative purposes we can use the case of a health promotion project to reduce alcohol consumption in a given locality. [Please note the example is used to highlight specific marketing/managerial issue rather than attempt to define an effective mental health promotion project.]

The first step in the process is to identify exactly what we want to achieve within the given resources i.e. the vision. As Confucius said,

For one who has no objectives nothing is relevant.

As the project develops the vision may be modified but only when discussed and agreed by the membership of the partnership. The vision focuses on the problem to be overcome or in a more positive mode, on the opportunities to be developed.

In this illustrative example the vision could be "to plan, develop and implement a programme to identify heavy and moderate drinkers and provide appropriate advice and support strategies to help individuals in each of the groups".

The next step is the identification of the project's overall objectives (Figure 1) which in turn leads to the identification of those parties (stakeholders) whose input and expertise is a prerequisite for a successful outcome.

Once the partnership of stakeholders is established the partnership has the task firstly to determine the specific tasks crucial to attainment of the project objectives and moving on from there, to allocate each of these specific tasks, by agreement, to the different stakeholder groups.

221

Figure 1: Identification of Overall Objectives

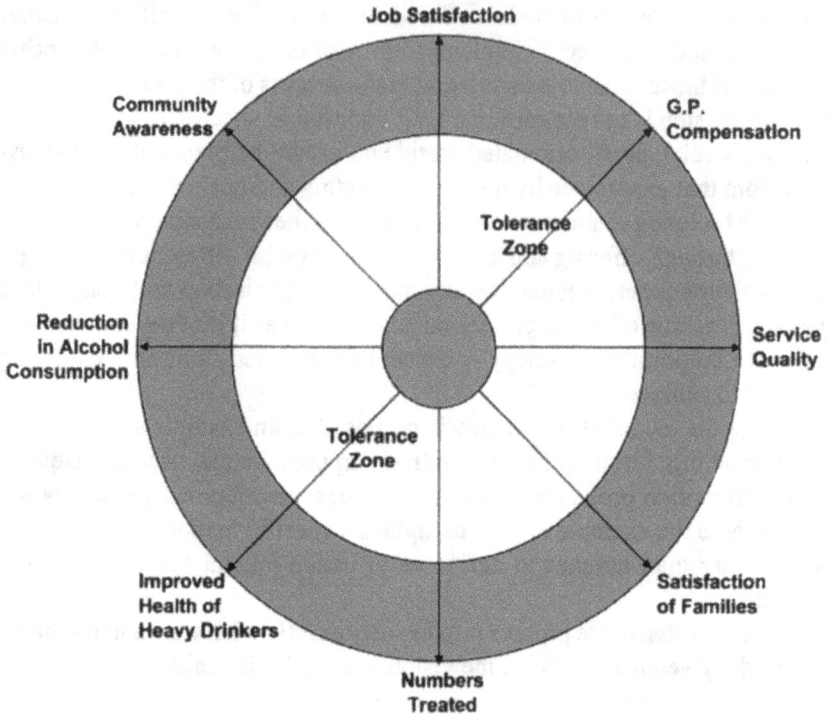

However to secure the commitment of the stakeholders in the partnership to the project it is important to identify and agree the "reward" for each of the stakeholder groups (see Figure 2) and then to reconcile any diverging and partly conflicting interests.

Conflicting rewards or aspirations are dealt with by bargaining and policy compromises to provide a societal grouping who work together to satisfy their separate interests. Bowman and Ash (1986), note that as long as every stakeholder group is satisfied with the relationship between its contribution to the project's effort and its rewards, the stakeholder coalition carries out its social and economic purpose.

In a well balanced organisation or project team reconciling these differences is not usually difficult as the different stakeholders do not usually seek to maximise their interests. Instead the stakeholder usually seeks "to gain a satisfactory return, expectations being based upon an incremental perspective of past rewards". The effective programme operates within the tolerance zone which is the band in which the programme is satisfying the interests of

222

Figure 2: Identifying the Reward for Stakeholders

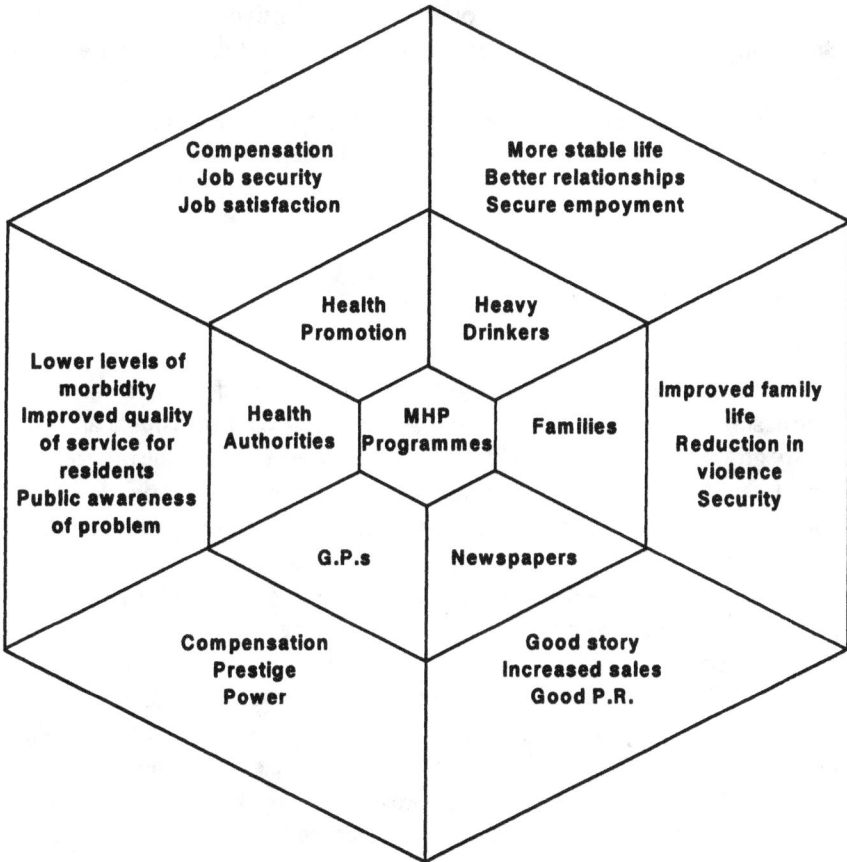

all its key stakeholders. As illustrated in Figure 1, when performance falls outside the tolerance zone the viability of the programme and the collaboration between the stakeholders is compromised. This is either because the programme fails to achieve minimum of performance or maximises exceptionally high levels of performance in some areas by minimising on others e.g. providing exceptionally high financial rewards for the general practitioners would mean minimising on another task that also require financial inputs. In summary we need to have both a balanced set of stakeholders and a balanced set of objectives.

To prevent the programme being captured by one group from among the different stakeholder groups it is essential that all the major stakeholders are fully represented at the highest level and so can participate fully in negotiating mutually agreed objectives and benefits for each of the groups. This is particularly important at the programme design stage when the vision and broad objectives are agreed and redefined into definite goals with specific measures of achievement to provide clear incentives for performance. Balancing the range of objectives means recognising that excellence is not likely to be achieved on a single measure. Maximising a specific objective today could lead to sacrificing other benefits tomorrow. The real task should be to achieve a satisfactory level of performance across a set of multiple, competing criteria.

Developing a Meaningful Partnership

Of course for such a model to be effective we need to develop meaningful partnerships between clinicians and mangers, between professional and voluntary groups and between health promoters and recipients of the programme objectives. By meaningful we mean the presence of a substantial degree of commitment from the different stakeholders, an understanding of each others roles and responsibilities in relation to the programme, the flexibility to accommodate each others differences in culture, background, expertise and political strength and a common recognition that there is strength in combining their diversity.

Because it is about relationships between different organisations the meaningful partnership demands trust and can only come about as a result of training, patience and the experience of working and learning together. Consequently there is no universal "correct" way to develop the partnership but the following essential ingredients need to be included;

a) Operational attitude and commitment
b) Shared vision and purpose
c) Agreed strategy, agreed targets and agreed performance goals
d) Clear roles and responsibilities
e) A fair risk/benefit ratio
f) Flexibility to take needs and views of the members into account
g) Clear commitment to the partnership in terms of resource and implementation
h) Ability for all to contribute to the decision making
i) Willingness to share power and information
j) Respect for each others differences.

Summary

The promotion of mental health is far too important to be left to the professionals. Mental health impinges on everyone and everyone has the right to be active in the promotion of their own mental health.

It is difficult to think of a logical argument against involving people in the promotion of their own mental health and yet there often appears reluctance to pursue this method of working. It is vital we seek ways to develop systems of working together to develop strategies to promote mental health and prevent mental disorders and the success or otherwise of work in this field will depend upon how well we are able to promote joint working between providing agencies and receivers of services.

References

Boone, L. E. and Kurtz D. L. (1992) *Contemporary Marketing Seventh Edition*, The Dryden Press, London.

Bowman, C. and Ash, D. (1986) *Strategic Management*, MacMillan Education Limited, London.

Doyle, P. (1994) *Marketing Management and Strategy*, Prentice Hall International (UK) Limited, Hemel Hempstead.

Kotler, P. (1991) *Marketing Management Analysis, Planning, Implementation and Control Seventh Edition*, Prentice Hall, Engelwood Cliffs, New Jersey.

MacDonald, T. H. (1998) *Rethinking Health Promotion A global Approach*, Routledge, London.

Morgan, G. (1997) *Images of Organization*, Sage, Thousand Oaks, California.

Schermerhorn, J. R. Jr., Hunt, J. G. and Osborn, R. N. (1997) *Organizational Behavior*, Wiley, New York.

Seedhouse, D. (1996) *Health Promotion Philosophy, Predudice and Practice*, Wiley, Chichester.

Simnett, I. (1997) *Managing Health Promotion: Developing Healthy Organisations and Communities*, Wiley, Chichester.

23 Socio-Cultural Adaptation and Social Support in Cross-Cultural Junior High School Classes

BRIT OPPEDAL

In this paper I will present findings from the initial screening of the research and development project "Interaction and Support in Multi-cultural Classes". The objective of the project is to examine the relations between selected individual and psychosocial variables and mental health among adolescents of Norwegian and Immigrant background, in a longitudinal perspective. The evaluation of interventions aimed at promoting social support among the students, is part of the study. The presented findings underline the importance of working with the psychosocial environment of the classroom to promote mental health among young adolescents, both of Norwegian and Immigrant origin. Social support from class will be seen in relation both to school problems and to socio-cultura marginalization. The risk and protective factors relevant to mental health in this study, can be described in the simplified model in Figure 1.

Research findings indicate a higher occurrence of mental health symptoms in different immigrant groups, both among children, adolescents and adults, compared to the majority population (Aronowitz, 1984). Researchers have tended to explain this variation based on either the "Selection hypothesis" stating a higher rate of people predisposed to mental problems among emigrants, or the "stress hypothesis" stating that the migration process is in itself promote psychological malfunctioning among immigrants/emigrants. Within the latter frame, variation in mental health has been analysed on the background of cultural differences, language proficiency, reason for migration, sojourn in host country and social status ambitions. (Böker, 1981, Cummins & Abdolell, 1981, Aronowitz, 1984, Parker & Kleiner, 1966, Dalgard &

Figure 1: Risk and Protective Factors Relevant to Mental Health in this Study

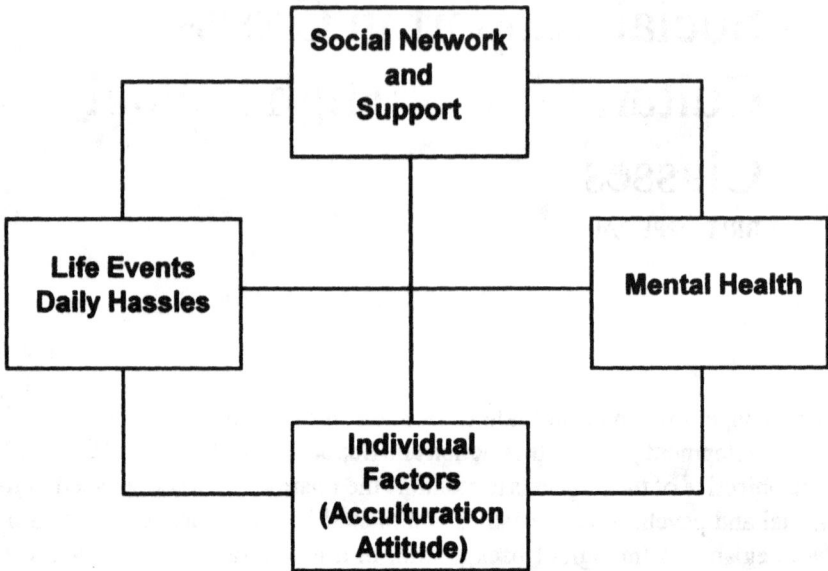

Døhlie, 1995). More recent studies among young immigrants, have also focused on the importance of differing socio-cultural attitudes and coping strategies to explain variations in psychological functioning. (Berry, 1989, Sam, 1994). Whereas strategies based on acceptance and respect for own cultural background (separation and integration) seem to be associated with psychological well-being, strategies that indicate rejection of ethnic heritage are related to psychological distress (assimilation and marginalization).

Findings from research examining the role of social support in adapting to stressful events during adolescence tend to show little consistency. Support has been found both for the direct and indirect (buffer) hypothesis on the effect of social support upon mental health, while other findings suggest that types and amount of both social support and stressors, may play different roles for males and females. (Rowlison. & Felner, 1988, Compas, Slavin, Wagner,. & Vannatta, 1996). Perceived social support also seems to be of importance for psychological adaptation in the migration process. (Murpy, 1973, Minde & Minde, 1976).

A pilot study at the upstart of this project, indicated differences in perceived social support from family and from classmates between Norwegians and Immigrants. Class support seemed to play an important role as a mediator in situations of school problems for both groups, and when Immigrant students report socio-cultural marginalization (Oppedal & Døhlie

228

1997). These findings provided the background for the intervention study targeting social support in the classroom.

Method

Subjects

Three hundred and ninety five students in 21 classes in 7 different junior high schools in Oslo, their teachers and the schools' psychologists participated in all of the project. Four hundred and fifty one students participated in the Time 1 screening half a year after up-start in junior high school, and 472 in the Time 2 screening a year later (about 85 % of all students). Thirty four per cent of the students are of Immigrant origin,(both parents come from another country than Norway) and 66 % of Norwegian (one or both parents of Norwegian background). The teachers and school psychologists were all of Norwegian origin. Informed consent from parents was required for the students to participate.

Design

The project has an experimental pre-test post-test design. The pre-and post-test is a questionnaire that the student and their teachers completed during two school lessons prior to and after the intervention. Help were given where language problems made answering difficult. This questionnaire serves various functions:

1) It gives information about factors influencing the students mental health.
2) It contributes necessary information to elaborate "The health profile of the class" which is the base of the interventions.
3) The survey also give a baseline for later evaluation of the effects of intervention and for analyses in a longitudinal perspective.

Measures

Mental health is in this project defined in terms of score on the Hopkin Symptom checklist, HSCL. This is a standardised scale, with scorerange from

1 - 4, measuring symptoms of anxiety, depression and somatizing. Scores > 1.75 are considered as high symptom level, suggesting that the distress might affect your everyday functioning.

Strain is measured in terms of negative life events related to acknowledged issues such as parents' divorce, their unemployment, health of self and others and «other events that I don't want to talk about». The more lasting hassles are related to school, family, and friends. "Goalstriving" represent the gap between obtained grades and the grades the students wish to obtain.

The quality of social support is measured by similar, but separate scales for family, friends, teachers and classmates. Scales' range from 1 (High level of support) to 3 (Low level). Class support has a cut-off point of 1.404 (median Norwegian students).

A scale developed on the basis of the theory of J.W. Berry and his colleagues is the basis for information on socio-cultural adaptation. The variables indicate degree of openness to own ethnic culture and that of the majority society. Scales on integration attitude and marginalization range from 1 (High preference) to 3 (Low preference) with cut-off score of 1.754.

Results

All students

Background differences
Of the Immigrants 43% are born in Norway, the mean sojourn for the rest of the group is 5.9 years (std. 3.6). Thirty five per cent have fathers from Pakistan, 10 % from Turkey and 6 % from Iran. 37 different countries are represented.

Of the Norwegian students, 38.2% have divorced or separated parents, compared to 18.5 % of the Immigrants (p=.000). Seventy point six per cent Immigrant and 3.8 % Norwegian adolescents report that religion is very important to them (p=.000). Twenty point five per cent Immigrants and 1.8% Norwegians, report that none of their parents are employed. In 46.4 % of the Immigrant and 82.7 % of the Norwegian families both parents are employed (p=.000).

Mental health
The average score on the HCSL 23 is 1.48. 63.5% of the students report a low degree of symptons, and 20.5% are in the "high degree of symptons" group. These findings are similar to those from other studies with

Norwegian high school students (Ystgaard, 1997).

In accordance with other studies, we find significant differences in mental health score between students of Norwegian and Immigrant background. (p=.003) with a higher rate of immigrant youth reporting more symptoms.

Strain: Negative life events and hassles

There are no significant differences between the two student groups in number of negative life events or hassles reported. But Norwegian students report more substance abuse problems among parents (p=.050), while immigrant students report higher incidence of unemployment/disablement benefit (p=.005) and academic problems (p=.021). This group also have higher level of goalstriving than their Norwegian schoolmates (p =.000). Except for goalstriving, there is significant correlation between number of life events and hassles related to school, family and friends on one hand and mental health on the other, both in the Immigrant and the Norwegian group.

Differences in social support

There are important differences between students with Norwegian and Immigrant background when we look at support from various social networks. While 59 % of the Norwegians report high level of class support, the percentage of Immigrants in the high level group is 48 (p= .037). A significant difference is also found in social support from family (p= .013), while the findings don't show differences in level of support from teachers and friends.

The correlation with mental health is significant for all 4 social support arenas, both for students of Norwegian and Immigrant origin. (Table 1).

Table 1: Correlations between different kinds of strain and mental health

	Life events	School problem	Family Problem	Friend problem	Goal-striving
Norwegian origin	.37***	.27***	.40***	-.30***	.08
Immigrant origin	.25**	.35***	.26**	-.29***	.13

*** p>.000, ** p>.001

The results of linear regressions for the two groups separately, to test the effect of social support from class on mental health, when controlled for strain and other support arenas, are presented in Table 2. The findings show that not only does class support contribute independently to variations in mental health. It is also the variable that contribute the most, both in the Immigrant and the Norwegian group. The family seems to be another important support arena, while the contribution from teachers and friends is non-significant under these circumstances.

Table 2: Linear regression analysis. Effect of social support on mental health, when controlled for strain

	Norwegians		Immigrants	
Negative life events	.223	.000	.071	.360
School related problems	.086	.097	.222	.005
Family related problems	.168	.003	.052	.514
Problems concerning friends	-.178	.000	-.073	.359
Support from class	.206	.000	.267	.002
Support from family	.146	.008	.213	.006
Support from teachers	.000	.993	-017	.825
Support from friends	.079	.149	.066	.388
	$R^2 = .38$	p=.000	$R^2=.34$	p=.000

The immigrant student and socio-cultural adaptation

One explicit goal of official Norwegian immigration policy, is socio-cultural integration. This is reflected in the School's Curriculum in different ways, and schools in areas with high density of immigrant students have become quite experienced in organising their teaching so that pupils from different cultures get to know and understand each other.

63 % of the Immigrant adolescents report high level of integration attitude, indicating that they favours an openness both to the culture of origin and to that of their new home country. On the other hand, 13 % report high level of marginalization. Integration attitude is positively, but not significantly, correlated with mental health, while marginalization shows significant negative correlation (p=.013). The findings also show a (very often significant) relation between integration attitude and positive outcome when different

problems and social support are concerned, while marginalization is (in many cases significantly) associated with negative outcome (Table 3).

Table 3: Correlations socio-cultural adaptation mental health, strain and social support

	Integration Attitude	Marginalis- ation
Mental Health	.157	-.200*
Life events	.097	-.166*
School problems	.170*	-.238**
Family problems	.222**	-.062
Problems related to friends	.181**	-.079
Goal striving	.069	-.076
Family support	.173*	-.384***
Class support	.267**	-.106
Teachers' support	.198*	-.087
Friends' support	.150	-.062

Direct or indirect effect of social support?

An often discussed issue within the social support research, is whether or not support is related to mental health independent of level of strain. To get information about whether the effect of class support is direct or indirect, separate analysis of interaction of class support and school problems were performed for the two groups. Interaction analysis was also done with class support and marginalization on behalf of the Immigrants students.

Unlike the findings from the pilot study, there are no implications for any buffer effect of class support when the students are under strain from school problems. But the implications for a direct effect of social support upon the mental health of both Norwegian and Immigrant students is apparent. When introducing the interaction variable into the analysis, the effect of school problems is no longer significant, while the main effect of class support is shown in a significance level of .01 for Norwegian and .000 for the Immigrant students.

The findings from similar analysis with an interaction variable made from marginalization with class support, has the same pattern. The significant effect of marginalization disappears when the interaction variable is introduced, while the direct effect of social support still is present. But may be the significance of the interaction variable of .079 still holds the door open for a possible indirect effect, had the sample been bigger.

Conclusion

The presented findings show that differences in social support seem to partly explain the differences in mental health between the students of majority and minority origin. Class support is the variable that explains most of the variance in mental health of adolescents of Immigrant and Norwegian origin.

In addition, positive experiences with classmates are associated with integration attitude to socio-cultural adaptation, while marginalization seems to be negatively related to these issues. Perception of belonging and being respected in a social network that is part of the "majority culture", like the school class obvious is, may be a necessary condition to develop the open-mindedness towards the host society which is important for successful socio-cultural integration.

The transition from primary school to junior high is hard on most students for many reasons. Higher expectations, strong increase in the theoretical approach to subjects, introduction of evaluation by means of grades and different teachers for different subjects. And while there is a heavy emphasis in primary school on the learning of social skills and creating good classroom environment, the emphasis in junior high is almost exclusively on subject matters. But taking into account the important association between class support and mental health, and between class support and socio-cultural integration, working on the classroom environment should be worth while also with older students. The fact that only slightly more than half of the adolescents report high level of support leaves a lot to be done!

References

Aronowitz, M. (1984) The social and emotional adjustment of immigrant children. A review of the literature. *International Migration Review,* 18 (2).

Berry, J.W. (1989) 'Psychology of Acculturation', in J. Berman (ed.) *Nebraska Symposium on Motivation 1989. Cross Cultural Perspectives,* Lincoln, Nebraska University Press.

Böker, W. (1981) 'Psycho(patho)logical reactions among foreign labourers in Europe', in L. Eitinger and D. Schwarz (eds.) *Strangers in the world,* Huber, 1981.

Compas, B. E., Slavin, L. A., Wagner, B. M. and Vannatta, K. (1986) *J. of Youth and Adolescence,* 15(3), pp. 205-221.

Cummins, J. and Abdolell, A. (1981) 'Bilingualism and educational adjustment of immigrant children: A case study of Lebanese families in Ontario' in L. Eitinger and D. Schwarz (eds.) *Strangers in the world,* Huber, 1981.

Dalgard, O. S. and Døhlie, E. (1995) 'Innvandring, sosiokulturell integrasjon og psykisk helse', in O. S. Dalgard, E. Døhlie and M. Ystgaard (eds.), *Sosialt nettverk, samfunn og helse.* Universitetsforlaget.

Minde, K. and Minde, A. (1976) Children of immigrants. *Canadian Psychiatric Association Journal,* 21.

Murphy, H. B. M. (1973) 'Migration and major mental disorders', in Zwingmann and Pfister-Ammende (eds.) New York, Springer, Berlin, Heidelberg,

Newcomb, M. D., Huba, G. J. and Bentler, P.M. (1981) A multidimensional assessment of stressful life events among adolescents: Derivation and correlates. *J. of Health and Social Behavior,* 22, pp. 400-415

Oppedal, B. and Døhlie, E. (1997) Betydningen av psykososiale miljøforhold i flerkulturelle klasser. *Rapport* 1/97.

24 Mental Health Promotion: Reflections on Future Challenges and Opportunities

MICHAEL KILLORAN-ROSS

In Great Britain, mental health promotion is in a period of transition. A movement that developed through a number of related fields, including Health Education and Community Development, and that, eventually, became explicitly aligned with and developed further through generic health promotion, is increasingly moving toward a distinct professional identity. Echoing the development of other professions in moving from the market place with apprenticeship training to the university with professional schools (Albee, 1998), there are now designated mental health promotion officers with specific remits in mental health promotion in most, if not all, health promotion departments throughout the United Kingdom. This is a relatively recent and positive change, but one that brings with it a range of difficulties. These difficulties appear most prominent in relation to the "core" identity of mental health promotion, the theory base on which it rests and the research methods it employs. These apparent difficulties will be explored in this paper.

In attempting to constitute a distinct core identity, a boundary appears to have been established, separating mental health promotion "specialists" from other people working in the area of mental health and/or community development. This has resulted in a kind of "ghettoisation" in which it has often appeared that mental health promotion specialists have actively sought to discourage participation from other disciplines. This exclusivity can be understood with reference to a number of constructs, including the paradigmatic framework first suggested by Burrell and Morgan (1979), in which intersecting relationships between theories of knowledge and theories of social control/social change were considered. The need for mental health promotion specialists, situated within the National Health Service, to define their identities and activities out with the prevailing medical model has been explained with reference to this framework. The difficulty with this exclusivity is that natural allies have often been repelled.

While understanding the need for mental health promotion specialists to define their practice outwith the medical model, it is also possible to suggest that this isolation is of little value to either the field of mental health promotion or to mental health service provision. The relationships between mental health service providers (Psychiatrists, Clinical Psychologists, Community Psychiatric Nurses, Counsellors) and Mental Health Promotion Specialists have often been, at best, fragile. For providers this may reflect the "functionalist" nature of their professions and may also reflect the frustration they feel in the current NHS climate. Faced with increasing demands for care and decreasing resources, it is, of course, understandable for service providers to argue that those resources that are available (both financial and human) should remain at the "coal-face" of treatment. Further, the effects of mental health promotion activities are seen in the long-term: while waiting for effects, providers continue to be overwhelmed with individual cases.

However, that status-quo will become increasingly untenable. In order for progress in mental health care, which both service providers and mental health promotion specialists must agree is the alleviation of preventable suffering for individuals, families and communities, the dialogue between service providers and mental health promotion specialists must be encouraged and shared solutions must be sought. (This ideal resolution is currently receiving impetus from central Government.) The facilitation of this dialogue is a "two-way street", in training and in practice, for both parties. For mental health promotion specialists, increased dialogue with providers (and others for whom mental health promotion is a priority issue) will ensure that work within the field moves more readily into the mainstream and out of its current status as "fringe activity". It must be noted that there are excellent examples of multi-disciplinary/ multi-agency working in Mental Health Promotion through-out the United Kingdom. However, these examples remain "models of good practice" rather than normative activities.

In developing the field of mental health promotion, clarification and explicit acknowledgement of the multi-disciplinary nature of the theory base on which practice evolves and depends must be sought. A number of commentators in the field have argued that mental health promotion exists almost as an isolated enclave, somewhat remote and detached from mainstream debates and developments in the social sciences (Mauthner, Ross and Brown, IN PRESS). Clearly, as there is potential for "ghettoisation" among mental health promotion specialists at the level of practice, so to, an isolationist mentality can occur at a theoretical level.

It may be that mental health promotion only exists in a coherent and inte-grated way, in its current construction as a profession, at the level of practice and that a distinct theoretical position is either temporarily unavailable or, indeed, may be ultimately impossible. Unfortunately, it appears that there is, at least on some occasions and in some settings, a belief that a value system, which informs model practice is, in fact, a theoretical basis for practice. It isn't: a value system is a value system, devised and supported by individuals in individual settings at specific periods of time. (This is not to deny the impor-tance of a value system in mental health promotion. Clearly, there is also a need to be explicit about those values which form the basis of the work and an examination of the current value system is, no doubt, part of the reflexivity that has been called for by practitioners in the field.) However, the confusion between theory base and value system has, it appears, been responsible for some of the excesses of "political correctness" in the field which have been unhelpful.

Research continues to be a vexed issue in mental health promotion. There appear to be several important difficulties with research in mental health pro-motion: apparently conflicting beliefs about research methodologies, a lack of coherence in research programmes, and, possibly as a result of the first two difficulties, a very real difficulty in demonstrating effectiveness for interven-tions from the promotion paradigm.

It appears, on some occasions, that a rather simplistic view about what constitutes "good" and "bad" research exists and that this view is polarised, often, by misunderstandings about both quantitative and qualitative research methodologies. It often appears, in the field of mental health promotion, that quantitative research is viewed as "bad" and qualitative research is viewed as "good". This dichotomy is far too simplistic to be of any utility and is a further example of the somewhat remote and detached relationship mental health pro-motion has with mainstream debates and developments in the social sciences. The issue of quantitative methods vs. qualitative methods in the social sciences is more-or-less resolved: even within the field of psychology, for example, where the randomised control trial, the testing of pre-conceived hypotheses on large samples randomly allocated to intervention and control conditions has historically been the "gold-standard" of research, there is increasing recogni-tion and acceptance of the vital importance of qualitative methods (Cooper and Stevenson, 1998). It appears obvious that the model of research employed must be appropriate to answer the underlying questions being asked; both methodologies are flawed, neither is necessarily intrinsically better than the other.

Qualitative approaches, which in very general terms, are concerned with

239

"...exploring, understanding and describing the personal and social experiences of participants and [with] trying to capture the meanings particular phenomena hold for [participants]...(Turpin, Barley, Beail, Scaife, Slade, Smith and Walsh, 1997) can be of particular value in the field, but only if the research is methodologically sound. In a recent comprehensive literature review, the inherent weaknesses in a significant proportion of the "research" in mental health promotion was demonstrated, and in many instances, research defined as qualitative was simply methodologically unsound research (Mauthner et al, IN PRESS).

There is an associated issue, particularly in Great Britain: the development and implementation of co-ordinated research programmes. Research is expensive and highly labour intensive. In our literature review, we observed the wide diversity of research undertaken in terms of subject areas (including a wide range of life events) participants (drawn from across most of the life stages) and settings (including, for example, the workplace, schools and a variety of community settings). In a sense, this variety is commendable. The difficulty, however, is that there has been little attempt to systematically map this activity in such a way that findings might inform training, policy or further research. Too often, it appears that where research is conducted, that research reflects the interests of an individual mental health promotion specialist and, possibly as a result, the major proportion of this research is person-centred.

There is a noticeable absence of research examining the interactive effects of people and social environments and for good reason: research in this area is much more difficult to design and, ultimately, to interpret in any meaningful way (Tilford, Delaney and Vogels, 1997). (However, this gap in the research base is a fundamental problem given the importance attached to environmental and structural factors in emotional well-being).

This "piece-meal" approach to research is exacerbated by the fact that those funding bodies awarding research money do not often include mental health promotion on their agendas and, although Health Authorities and Health Boards are increasingly conscious of the necessity of including mental health promotion within appropriate strategy documents, they have not, as yet, appeared to understand the importance of commissioning appropriate research in the field.

There is an obvious need for co-ordinated national and inter-national research programmes in mental health promotion. This goal should be achievable; perhaps not easily achievable, but achievable. In Great Britain, the basic concept of co-ordinated research strategy has been accepted by funding bodies and researchers in other areas of health care (The Scottish Office, 1998). At previous conferences in this series, there have been calls for both more multi-centre trials and the replication of model programmes across national boundaries. It may be that the Clifford Beers Foundation has roles to play both in lobbying for the establishment of National Research Programmes and/or in the co-ordination of existing research trials within the United Kingdom.

As a small step in the direction of co-ordinating research programmes, the Scottish Needs Assessment Programme (SNAP), which, as the title would suggest, is responsible for making appropriate recommendations to Scottish Health Boards on the basis of National needs assessment, commissioned work on mental health promotion among young people aged 12-18 years. Our work in the group is about to go to consultation with a variety of stakeholders and among our recommendations will be specific recommendations for research which, once implemented by Health Boards, will provide a co-ordinated model for research strategy among this population. Work with other populations might generate similar cohesive research strategies. Clearly, by co-ordinating research efforts, there is a greater likelihood of progress being achieved.

Conclusion

There is no compelling reason to believe that emotional distress and/or mental disorder is going to decrease. In fact, recent evidence suggests that the opposite appears more likely and there is a very real need for mental health promotion. However, we can only meet that need by, in a sense, "getting our own shops in order." If we can achieve that aim, then our contribution, our very real contribution, can be successfully made.

References

Albee, G.W. (1998). Fifty years of clinical psychology; Selling our soul to the devil. Applied and Preventive Psychology (7). 189-194.

Burrell. G. & Morgan, G. (1979). Sociological paradigms and organisational analysis. London: Heinemann.

Cooper, N. & Stevenson, C. (1998). 'New science' and psychology. The Psychologist (11) 484-485.

Mauthner, N., Ross, M.K. & Brown, J. (In Press). Mental Health Promotion Theory and Practice; Insights From a Literature Review.

The Scottish Office (1998). Research Strategy for the National Health Service in Scotland.

Tilford, S., Delaney, F. & Vogels, M. (1997). Effectiveness of mental health promotion intervenitons: a review. London: Health Education Authority.

Turpin, G., Barley, V., Beail, N., Scaife, J., Slade, P., Smith, J.A., Walsh, S. (1997). Standards for research projects and theses involving qualitative methods: suggested guidelines for trainees and courses. Clinical Psychology Forum (108) 3-7.

25 Developing Respectful Relationships With Young People Through Mental Health Promotion: Youth Partnership Accountability[1]

KATHLEEN STACEY[2]

Abstract

In Western societies, adults make the rules, set the standards, determine priorities and criteria, judge value, appropriateness and relevance, control resources and administer consequences. This is apparent in the policies and practices of the mental health field where adults take responsibility for determining the realities of young people's lives and intervening in accordance with these determinations. In conversations between mental health workers and young people, language can be a place of struggle. Meanings are often constructed about young people's life circumstances which may not fit with their lived experience.

Mental health promotion projects that adopt a community development approach endeavour to develop respectful relationships with the target group. When the focus is young people, this means engaging in youth participation. *Youth partnership accountability* is a very respectful and enabling approach to youth participation through which young people have significant direction and control over a project. This paper will describe some elements of *youth partnership accountability* in transforming relationships between adults and young people in the context of the successful CHAMPS rural youth mental health promotion project (Community Health Adolescent Murraylands Peer Support).

Introduction

Remembering: "As you drive down the last hill and turn off the freeway into Murray Bridge[3] to start work, you ponder the features of this rural area: Murray Bridge is an hour from the city, but at times a world away; high unemployment; one of the lowest income/capita areas in the country; no public transport outside Murray Bridge; entrenched racism affecting the Indigenous population; large areas of public housing; resentment from old Murray Bridgites of the public housing population; no dedicated youth emergency accommodation; elevated school dropout rates; strong homophobia; limited community services, ranging to almost non-existent in the outlying areas; an overstretched child welfare service; a strong sport and alcohol culture; no youth recreation area; isolation in the outlying areas.

It doesn't seem such a surprise that staple issues brought to your community-based therapy service are the effects of abuse and violence, depression and suicide, nor that the demand for your services far outweighs your capacity to respond. You know that you are seeing the tough face of poverty, racism, sexism and the effects of dominant societal structures on young people, along with the vicissitudes of life that we all face and for which we all need support. A gloomy picture, a hard grind in the activity trap, "life-saving" efforts as you fish people out of the river so they don't drown - many of us remain in this mode. However, another vision emerged that went beyond the efforts to achieve community participation and accountability to the community that your team had tried thus far."

CHAMPS: Visions and Intentions

Enabling 13-18 year youth in the Murray-Mallee region to have a voice in shaping the way in which mental health services are provided to them and to participate in mental health promotion activities became the goal of the grant funded CHAMPS project which commenced in early 1996.

The initial vision was for the development of Youth Forums, meeting up to 8 times/year and consisting of around 12 young people (this immediately grew to 25-30!), which identified the mental health needs of their peers, how they wished agencies/adults to work effectively with their peers and communities and how they could promote mental health amongst their peers. Secondly, there was the establishment of Youth Access and Resource Network (YARN) to enable young people to talk to other young people in a peer support framework by telephone. It soon became apparent we were also creating a model of best practice for working in partnership with young people.

Intentions for the project included to:

- create a sense of connection between young people across the large rural region of the Murray-Mallee,
- include those young people who are not always chosen as representatives i.e. not necessarily prominent school members or members of Student Representative Councils, but those who are not in school and young people from different cultural backgrounds,
- work in a way which is more demanding of adults,
- provide an experience for young people that sought to be respectful, empowering and possibly fairly novel,
- acknowledge the skills, knowledges and experiences of young people and the resource they can be to each other in supporting their emotional well-being.

CHAMPS was based on the philosophy and practice of Youth Partnership Accountability, primary health care and health promotion principles (World Health Organisation, 1986), social justice and practices of inclusion. Thus, adults were in positions of support in relation to young people and were accountable to young people for their actions, a whole of population focus and holistic approach to mental health were taken and efforts were made to transcend barriers of distance and difference for young people. At every turn of the project, whether it was in determining the role of the CHAMPS Forums, setting priorities for action, designing elements of mental health promotion projects, strategising about the future of CHAMPS or designing the evaluation process, there has been a committed endeavour to live out the philosophy of Youth Partnership Accountability.

Adult Challenges in Developing Respectful Relationships with Young People

Partnership, along with empowerment, are key concepts within primary health care and health promotion rhetoric, especially within community development approaches. However, it has been noted that slippage from "empowerment" into "coercion" can occur, however benevolent, and the accountability component of partnership often receives less explicit attention or commentary (Wass, 1994).

Partnership Accountability is an outgrowth of postmodern influences within both therapeutic and community development fields that examines the social-political implications of engaging in such work (eg Hall, 1994; McLean, 1994; Tamasese & Waldegrave, 1993). *Youth Partnership Accountability* (YPA) is an approach through which adults support young people in creating preferred realities in their lives (Black, 1995; Black & McLean, 1995; Stacey, 1998a; 1998b).[4] It can be practised in one-to-one therapeutic relationships through to group and community projects. YPA in mental health promotion means young people construct meanings that fit their lived experiences and adults respond to and support them in designing ways of promoting mental health based on these meanings and an understanding of the contextual and structural influences on young people's lives.[5]

Principles and Practices of Youth Partnership Accountability Include (Stacey, 1997)

- sharing of decision-making powers between service providers and young people,
- service providers preventing exploitation of young people's time, energy and ideas by themselves or others,
- service providers and funding bodies acknowledging young people's contributions (including payment of travel costs, expenses and time given),
- service providers having a willingness to be flexible,
- service providers having a commitment to seeing young people as *persons,* rather than young people losing their sense of personhood by service providers collapsing young people's identities into the problems in their lives,
- service providers involving young people in as many aspects of service design and delivery as possible,
- young people having the right to say no and have choice about services, which includes service providers being clear they are giving permission for this and acting with integrity when this occurs,
- service providers acknowledging the wider social-political contexts of young people's lives,
- service providers ensuring accessibility of services,
- ongoing dialogue between service providers and service receivers, and service providers demonstrating transparency, both professionally and personally.

Accountability becomes the crucial key in determining whether YPA is part of young people's lived experience. Instead of decentring ourselves and

246

just focusing on young people, adults need to center themselves in the process. This is not from an expert position, "I am an authority on young people and my view predominates," but from a position of critical reflection and consciousness (Freire, 1970; 1994), "what effects do my beliefs and actions have on young people and do these effects contribute positively to their lives." This places adults in an ethical position, although one that may challenge some predominant ethical notions for workers. This means engaging with the dynamics of power and privilege described in the first paragraph of the abstract.

It has been proven that good will and a desire to learn is not always enough because questions emerge such as: on whose terms, whose opinions are more important or accurate and who is respected as a valued teacher rather than just a handy resource (Black, Gale, Hills, Moulds, Stacey, Stone, Tully & Webb, 1998). If the answers to these questions are not young people/youth consultants, then issues of power on which accountability rest need to be examined (Stacey, 1998a; Stacey & Turner, 1998).

Youth Partnership Accountability Within the Context of CHAMPS

Black (1995) has stated,

> As adults, we can't decide what partnerships with youth will look like. We need to ask them if it is actually something they want. We need to ask ourselves is it something that we are putting upon young people, and by doing this replicating the oppression of young people. We need to hear young people's ideas and motivations and take the trip together. (p.43)

Taking the trip together is crucial, as is accepting that making mistakes along the way is grist for the mill for both adults and young people. What counts, particularly as the adult, is how you recover the mistakes, how transparent you are about their existence and your responsibility for them. In CHAMPS, we had a practice of letting young people know when we believed we had made a mistake, responding respectfully and humbly when they informed us of a mistake or, where possible, calling ourselves on something before they did. Too often, people in the less powerful position of the partnership have the responsibility of calling the more powerful to account which perpetuates a sense of having to beg for respect, rather than it being seen as their right. The difference that dealing openly with mistakes can make is illustrated through an excerpt from the January 1998 evaluation interview of

247

CHAMPS project staff. An event that occurred while at an interstate conference with young people was being discussed:

Kathleen: ... even when things get tough, and there's several times when things have got tough in relationships with young people, and a couple of times they didn't work out so well, and then there were other times when they could have been absolutely bloody disastrous and they weren't. In fact we came out on the other side closer and better friends. I was talking to one of the CHAMPS recently and we were laughing about an experience that was actually really hard for us at one of the conferences. Now we think its just such an enormous joke. I talked with him quite honestly about my worries that I did the right thing at the time and what it was like for me in the middle of the night to be woken up with this request and how I hadn't taken it seriously until I got off the phone and thought, "Oh fuck, they're serious. I'd better go find them"...

Cindy: I think that what you're talking about is when someone wanted to basically challenge the very few rules...

Kathleen: Well we didn't even call them rules, they were agreements.

Cindy: But they challenged it in a way where they actually came...

Kathleen: To me and said, "I'm challenging this and will you help me out with challenging it," and I'm going, "This is a dilemma for me. I can't support you to challenge this because I know the consequence of you challenging this, is that the next day I'll be saying, "I'm sorry matey, but this is the agreement and everyone agreed and you've got to go home!"

Leanne: And the dilemma is, if you don't engage with what that request is, then it has a consequence too.

Cindy: And you lose that person too.

Leanne: And you put that person at risk in some way.

Kathleen: Yeah, this is what I was talking about with this CHAMPS member who was involved, although he wasn't the person I'm talking about now [who did the direct challenging]. He said, "He really trusted you." And I said, "Yeah, that's what I took it as. I took that as an enormous compliment," because as this CHAMPS member said, "That's not something he'd ever ask his mother."

Cindy: But then there was also that sense that because the answer had been no, the answer was no because you wouldn't be safe and so that was actually OK. So, well, yes, it was "I trusted you and that trust was validated because you looked after my safety. You didn't look after just saying yes to be nice people."

Kathleen: I think what I did was I got off the phone and then realised there was a risk here and that he'd asked for me to provide some safety for him and I'd said no to that piece of safety because I was looking after the rest of his safety. But if I hadn't gone and found him I wouldn't have actually looked after the rest of his safety, so I wanted to do that.

Leanne: You said to me only a couple of weeks ago [something] that's really kept me thinking about this, its youth partnership **and** accountability. The accountability is the bit that actually makes your youth partnership stay together and keep on flowing. The accountability bit has us being stuck often, or challenged to know which next bit, which next direction, how? These are just ideas, the partnership stuff about philosophy and respect, the accountability is "Well, how we get to **do** that as adults, with our own whole lot of stuff and training and whatever? How do we sift through that when we have to act and have to make a decision just like that?"

Kathleen: I think this is what's critical for workers to know going into this work, because I think there's a lot of rhetoric around partnership. People sort of feel that its not so hard to do, although they don't always know how to do it...

Leanne: But that's not the most radical concept either.

Kathleen: No, its not. It's the accountability, because that means if you screw up, you have to say you did and you have to do something about it.

Leanne: And you actually have to realise it.

Kathleen: You have to realise it, you have to do something about it, and you have to say that to someone you normally don't think you have to say that to, because you're in a position of power over them.

Leanne: In fact you might have to go a step further and work out a way for them to let you know whether you've stuffed up.

Kathleen: Exactly, because they probably won't tell you. So a way of constantly checking, so it becomes a normal thing, is to always **check** with them and show that we're willing to hear. So when they actually need to say it, they know that its not a foreign idea to us either, because we've laid this foundation through saying, "If we do something that's not OK, its really important to tell us," or we would try and give an example like, "Oh I got that wrong," or whatever and so we'd have the language present during forums and during other times where we'd acknowledge that we didn't do things quite right. Or we'd come to them and say, "We took this step and we realised we didn't ask you. We actually feel quite badly about this, but this is why we found ourselves taking this step."

There are many other important features to the practice of YPA which have been and will continue to be articulated (Black, 1995; Black, et al, 1998; Black & McLean, 1995; Stacey, 1997; 1998a; 1998b; 1998c; Stacey & Turner, 1998). A detailed account of CHAMPS work is beyond the scope of this paper, but can be found in Stacey (1997) and Stacey & Turner (1997; 1998).

The Achievements of CHAMPS

CHAMPS far exceeded its initial expectations, in terms of anticipated outcomes held by both Project Staff and young people in CHAMPS, and spawned **many** peer designed mental health promotion projects, including:

- CHAMPS by the River, a youth designed youth-friendly recreation area in Murray Bridge.
- CHAMPS Camp, which incorporated extensive planning for CHAMPS projects.
- Media Liaison, where young people write for and/or participate in media activities.
- YARN peer support phone service.
- Youth Week activities held in State Youth Week, Sept '97, including the opening of CHAMPS by the River.
- CHAMPS Youth Art, free workshops to promote youth art and prepare a piece of public youth art at the CHAMPS by the River Art Wall.
- The Rage Cage, a sporting facility consisting of a court designed for a variety of ball sports and skating in a safe youth friendly environment as an addition to CHAMPS by the River.
- Consultations for government, other agencies and community groups.

250

- Conference presentations at eight conferences, both national and international.
- Intersectoral collaboration with other agencies and sectors.
- "Talking Together: Young People Educating Adults" Inaugural CHAMPS conference to educate adult health, welfare, educational workers and community members on youth friendly practice, the principles of youth partnership accountability and discuss the community's commitment to supporting a sustainable future for CHAMPS.

Further, it garnered intersectoral support to ensure continued funding and has gained a local building to establish a regional youth centre. CHAMPS has been extensively evaluated, both during and at the end of its first two years of operation, involving all key stakeholders. Overall, CHAMPS has been perceived as a very successful project that lived up to its intention of establishing a best practice model for working in partnership with young people and comprehensively met all its objectives. The overwhelmingly consistent outcomes have been:

- the need for CHAMPS to be ongoing in the Murraylands,
- the recommendation that programs like CHAMPS be made available in other areas of South Australia, and
- the endorsement of youth partnership accountability as a highly recommended approach to working with young people which enables them to not only have a voice on concerns central to their lives, but be responded to by adults and workers in respectful ways.

Conclusion

Mental health promotion with young people is, potentially, a pathway to preferred futures. YPA is an important means by which such potentiality can come to fruition. YPA builds on solid foundations in mental health promotion philosophy and practice, yet extends it through open acknowledgment of power and privilege vis a vis adults and young people.

References

Black, L. (1995) "Youth Partnership: An exploration of the power relations between adults and young people", *Family Therapy Association of South Australia Newsletter*, Summer, pp. 39-43.

Black, L., Gale, K., Hills, S., Moulds, D., Stacey, K., Stone, P., Tully, D. & Webb, E. (1998) *Workshop report - "Working relationships with young people: What about power?."* Youth SA., Adelaide.

Black, L. & McLean, C. (1995) 'Working with young people in a context of equity: A conversation with Leanne Black', *Dulwich Centre Newsletter*, Nos 2 & 3, pp. 90-94.

Freire, P. (1970) *Pedagogy of the Oppressed*, Continuum, New York.

Freire, P. (1994) *Pedagogy of hope: Reliving "Pedagogy of the oppressed."* Continuum, New York.

Hall, R. (1994) Partnership accountability, *Dulwich Centre Newsletter*, Nos 2 & 3, pp. 6-29.

McLean, C. (1994) A conversation about accountability with Michael White, *Dulwich Centre Newsletter*, Nos 2 & 3, pp. 68-79.

Tamasese, K. & Waldegrave, C. (1993) 'Cultural and gender accountability in the "Just Therapy" approach', *Journal of Feminist Family Therapy*, 5;2, pp. 29-45.

Stacey, K. (1997). 'Breathing life into youth partnership: "We come together, to talk things over and work things out", in J. Toumbourou, M. Carr-Gregg and F. Sloman (eds.), *Harnessing Peer Influence in Adolescent Health Promotion*, Centre for Adolescent Health Monograph Series, Melbourne.

Stacey, K. (1998a) 'Accountability: The forgotten aspect of youth partnership accountability', *Health Promotion Quarterly*, February, pp. 3-4.

Stacey, K. (1998b) *Youth partnership accountability: Creating preferred realities with young people.* Paper presented at the 3rd Biennial Conference of the Discursive Production of Knowledge Group: "Postmodernism in Practice," Adelaide, Feb 24 - Mar 1, 1998.

Stacey, K. (1998c) *Theoretical underpinnings of youth partnership accountability.* Paper presented at the "Working relationships with young people: What about power?" workshop, Adelaide, May 8, 1998.

Stacey, K. & Turner, C. (eds.) (1997) *Talking together: Young people Educating Adults*, Proceedings of the Inaugural CHAMPS Project Conference, November 11, 1997, Murray Bridge, South Australia, Southern CAMHS, Adelaide.

Stacey, K. & Turner, C. (1998) *The CHAMPS Project: Evaluation Report*, Southern CAMHS, Adelaide.

Wass, A. (1994) *Promoting health: The primary health care approach*, Harcourt Brace & Co., Sydney.

World Health Organisation, (1986) *Ottawa charter for health promotion*. Ottawa, Canada: World Health Organisation, Health and Welfare Canada and the Canadian Public Health Association. Also published in the 1987, 1(4) edition of *Health Promotion*, pp. i-v.

Acknowledgements

This work is only possible through the enthusiasm, goodwill, commitment and generosity of young people who engage in such projects. I co-write work with CHAMPS members when we can, but this has not happened on this occasion although they are aware of the paper. Thanks also to Cindy Turner, my valued co-traveller for 2 years in CHAMPS, who became Project Coordinator when I left that position in early 1998.

Appendix A

In our society, it is adults who have most of the say about what happens to people. They make the decisions about lots of things in young peoples' lives. Sometimes these are helpful decisions, sometimes they are not. Many times, adults make decisions without checking how young people feel or what they think about them.

If adults talked more with young people about decisions that have to be made, really listened to young people and used their ideas, this would mean they are trying to work in partnership with young people. Partnership is about doing things together. It is about listening to everyone's voice and taking different ideas seriously - even when they don't make sense at first. It is about mutual respect. It is about adults explaining what decisions have to be made and working out how to make them with young people [as well as young people explaining to adults what decisions they believe need to be made].

Partnership is about adults explaining why they choose to do the things they do, especially when these actions effect young people. It is about adults hearing what effect their actions have on young people, both the good effects and the bad effects. It is about adults taking responsibility for finding ways of preventing bad effects and working with young people to find out how to do this. Partnership is about adults giving young people all the support they need so they can participate in making decisions about their lives or working on projects that effect young people.

Partnership is about seeing young people as people, sometimes as people who have problems in their lives, but not seeing young people as problems to be solved. It is about being flexible. It is about knowing that young people have important contributions to make about decisions that effect their lives. Partnership also means both adults and young people working hard (Stacey, 1997, p.35).

253

Notes

1   Based on a workshop presented at the 8th Annual European Conference on the Promotion of Health, Birmingham, UK, 10th September, 1998.
2   Program Coordinator, Graduate Programs in Community Mental Health, Department of Public Health, Flinders University, South Australia and CHAMPS Project Consultant. *Address*: c/- Southern CAMHS, The Flats, Flinders Medical Centre, Bedford Park, SA 5042, Australia.
3   Murray Bridge is a rural city of ~13,000 people in South Australia, 80kms east of Adelaide. It is the identified regional centre for a rural district or ~25,000 people extending .5 hours west, 1.5 hours drive north, 2 hours east and 1 hour south, made up of small towns, farming districts and isolated farms.
4   Developing appropriate language for each context is important as the adult or adult worker/young person distinction does not always fit. Some workers are still young people (ie 25 years or under) so the term youth consultant can be helpful.
5   A youth-friendly version of YPA is contained in Appendix 1. An overview of the theoretical basis of YPA can be found in Stacey (1998c).

26 Mental Health Promotion Within the Primary School Setting - Lanarkshire's Experience

GRAEME WALSH

1. Introduction and Background

1.1 Background

The Health Promotion Department, Lanarkshire Health Board, in partnership with North and South Lanarkshire Councils, introduced a mental health promotion initiative into local primary schools to coincide with Scottish Mental Health Week and World Mental Health Day 1997.

There were two parts to the initiative:

- A half price admission voucher to a Council leisure amenity. This was aimed at encouraging the child to invite their parent(s) or guardian to spend time together. The voucher was circulated to all children at participating primary pchools.
- The schools who participated in the initiative could select one of nine options targeted at dealing with mental health issues. The objective was for the Health Board to provide appropriate support material which the school could use to integrate into curriculum activities. The options included a variety of activities targeted at the children, however additional options were available for parents and/or teachers.

The following options were provided in relation to children activities:

- Healthy Eating Roadshow;

- exercise - Fitness Team;
- self esteem - Structured Play;
- Playground Games Pack;
- Playground Marking;
- Self Esteem Builder Pack.

The following options were targeted at parents and teachers:

- reflexology;
- aromatherapy;
- Tai Chi;
- relaxation techniques.

Schools were informed of the initiative through the internal mail system used by the Education Department. The information pack contained an order form with a two page summary of the options available. This information was circulated to all Lanarkshire primary schools in September 1997. Having identified participating schools, the admission vouchers were then sent to the Head Teachers prior to Mental Health Week in October.

2. Survey Method

Qualitative research was implemented and a programme of school visits were arranged. At each school visit an in-depth interview was conducted with the Head Teacher (or nominated teacher who was liaison for the initiative). Depending on the size of the school, up to two other teachers were interviewed. Where possible, with the schools' permission, pupils were also interviewed. All interviews were conducted by Senior Consultants from Axiom Market Research & Consultancy.

In designing the interview schedule cognizance was taken of the following issues:

- an equal split between North and South Lanarkshire Council schools;
- inclusion of a special needs school in both Council areas;
- inclusion of the rural view in both Council areas;
- teachers responsible for teaching pupil of different age groups (Primary 1-3, Primary 4-5 and Primary 6-7);
- a sample of pupils within Primary 1-3, 4-5 and 6-7.

The in-depth interviews followed a semi-structured discussion guide which was designed and agreed with the Working Group at Lanarkshire Health Board.

The following sample was interviewed in the first two weeks of December:

- 7 Head Teachers;
- 7 Teachers;
- The South Lanarkshire Heads of Small Schools Forum (representing the rural view in South Lanaarkshire);
- Pupils in:
    2 Primary 1-3 classes;
    2 Primary 4-5 classes;
    2 Primary 6-7 classes.

The breakdown of schools included two special needs schools (one in each Council area), a rural school in North Lanarkshire and four urban schools, (two in each Council area).

3. Summary of Findings

3.1 Reaction to the Initiative

Having participated in the initiative, the schools believed that it was appropriate to begin to raise awareness of mental health issues within the primary school setting. However, it is interesting to note that schools use different language when discussing the issues, compared to LHB . The Teachers do not use the phrase "mental health" - they refer to it as "healthy living", although clearly the core issues are the same. Indeed, the issues are clearly identified in the National Curriculum Guidelines covering Personal and Social Development and Environmental Education.

3.2 Support Material

Consideration was given to the appropriateness of the various options which were available to the schools. There was wide support for the child related options. Indeed, schools responded particularly well to two options:

- Healthy Eating Roadshow;
- Playground Marking.

First reaction suggested that all options were considered to be appropriate. However, further discussion revealed that while all options were considered useful, only the 'child related' options were considered to be of *value* as they closely met the needs of the school.

There was particularly strong support for the Healthy Eating Roadshow, as this ties into the school curriculum across all ages. Indeed, there are a number of ways in which healthy eating is discussed within the schools. Younger pupils work on a project basis to identify healthy foods. Catering Direct also have an initiative known as 3-2-1, and some schools have particular healthy eating days at meal times.

Therefore the Healthy Eating Roadshow was an option that was in line with other work being done in the schools. Furthermore, the concept of a guest speaker visiting the school and conducting a presentation was extremely well liked as it appears to offer a number of advantages. From the pupils' perspective, somebody new in the classroom gives the message an extra dimension which seems to improve their recall of events and therefore underlines the message. Secondly, from the teachers' perspective, the event is extremely easy to arrange and can easily be slotted into classroom activities at short notice.

A number of the schools visited had already benefited from the Healthy Eating Roadshow. The feedback was extremely positive as the visits appear to have been tailored to meet the needs of the school. One topic considered to be particularly useful included 'Making up a healthy pack Lunch Box'. However, it is worth commenting that one teacher suggested that this is the type of event that both child and parent would benefit from.

Another key area considered important to the children's development is that of active play. There seems to a very strong concern amongst teachers that this aspect of school life needs to be improved. Teachers recognise the importance of structured play in not only improving fitness but also developing positive behaviour and building relationships. Consequently, the Playground Games Pack and Playground Marking options proved very popular.

Some of the schools interviewed had received the Playground Games pack, but not all had immediately made use of the information. One school was integrating the pack into class work by developing a Primary Seven project around the material. Another school had not made use of the Pack as it was the wrong time of year and would review the information in the Spring. However, a Head Teacher indicated that schools were inundated with similar packs, such as the Scottish Football Association's 'Super Striker' Pack.

As the teachers have to read the material, then plan an effective action, the usefulness of the pack is reduced due to constraints in terms of the teachers' time. Whilst all teachers interviewed appear to have the needs of the children in mind, they all mentioned a constant pressure at work indicating a lack of time to do all the things that they would like to do.

The Playground Marking Pack proved to be extremely popular. As one school indicated, this type of pack would always be needed as markings tend to fade and always need replaced. Furthermore, any additional resources that encourage active play is considered to be beneficial.

Promoting positive behaviour support material was considered important but proved less popular, as Teachers believed that positive behaviour would result from active and structured play. Therefore teachers believed the emphasis should be on encouraging active play, particularly at break times.

Teachers recognised the benefits of the Managing Self options, but they did not prove to be as popular. Teachers believe the emphasis should be on meeting the children's needs. Furthermore, schools were aware that such activities were available through other sources such as HEBS (Health Education Board for Scotland). This is an interesting point revealing a lack of awareness of the role of LHB. However, as Head Teachers are more budget orientated, the confusion appears to arise as the application for funding is made to HEBS.

Teachers also commented that it is important to get parents involved, but were surprised that none of the options included parent and child participating in an event together (although they did recognise that this was the objective behind the admission voucher).

Another issued raised was that some interviewees had reservations regarding the 'Managing Self' options. Indeed, one interviewee commented that there had recently been a directive from the Education Department outlining that care should be taken when identifying individuals to participate in such events. Therefore there appeared to be some confusion over the suitability of the Managing Self options.

Teachers were asked to identify other options that they would like to see if the initiative is repeated. Most suggested that Managing Self options should be replaced, and forwarded the following ideas where parents and child could participate:

- Line Dancing (including music and dance step material);
- Scottish Dancing (including music and dance step material);
- aerobics classes conducted in the school.

In principle, the teachers supported the issue of the voucher, as they could see that the Admission Voucher supported the Healthy Living message within the school curriculum. They could also appreciate that the voucher would encourage parents and children to spend quality time together.

However, there appears to have been an extremely low uptake of the vouchers. The pupils were asked if they could remember receiving the voucher and if they had used them. Findings from the straw poll, although not statistically valid, indicated that typically a quarter of pupils remembered receiving the leaflets and only a handful had actually used the voucher.

As a result, the voucher does not appear to have been a catalyst in encouraging repeat usage at the Council Leisure facilities. It is worth commenting that teachers recognised the importance of improving access to leisure facilities from the children's perspective as new activities help in the child's development. They also recognised the importance to the Council's Leisure Department to attract new customers at a young age to improve levels of usage.

Upon further discussion, a number of significant problems emerged with the voucher scheme. These primarily related to the way in which the vouchers were circulated within the school. The Head Teachers were asked to inform teachers about the voucher. The teacher would then pass the vouchers to the children within class. The child would the keep the voucher all day and give it to their parent or guardian on returning home. However, feedback suggests that it was not uncommon for the children to "bin them or make paper planes out of them".

There were also examples of the Head Teacher stating that they had briefed the teachers and that the leaflets had been circulated. However, when interviewed, neither the teachers nor the children could remember receiving the voucher.

Alternative distribution was discussed during the interviews, and a number of ideas were forwarded. These included using the Parents Teachers Association or school newsletters, which are sent directly to the parent.

It was felt that working with the Parents Teachers Association would not impact upon the type of parent that would benefit most from the voucher. Therefore the distribution wouldn't reach the target audience.

The use of the school newsletter would have a better chance of reaching the right audience. However, it appears that not all schools produce a regular school newsletter. Furthermore, the schools would require support to meet the operational cost and involvement of producing and circulating the newsletter. Once again, some teachers had reservations about whether such a course of action would impact on parental involvement.

There is also the question of cost effectiveness, as teachers recognise that the school newsletter is regarded as 'junk mail' when it is sent directly to the household.

The interviews revealed that teachers believed the vouchers to be orientated towards middle income families in urban areas. The view of rural schools was similar, with comments suggesting that some rural facilities (swimming pool) had been omitted from the voucher scheme. Furthermore, the issue of accessibility arose. North Lanarkshire suffers from poor public transportation links to some of the facilities. Indeed residents are more likely to use facilities in the Kirkintilloch area. South Lanarkshire respondents also commented on poor accessibility to key facilities and indicated that using public transport was cost prohibitive.

Although the voucher offered half price admission, it was still the teachers' opinion that the price of an excursion to a leisure facility would be cost prohibitive for many low income families.

Another issue that arose was in relation to the timing of the voucher. The voucher was to be used during Mental Health Week, which was a fortnight after the school holiday. Consequently, many respondents suggested that this be linked to the holiday period. Further discussion revealed that this opinion related to the feeling that parents would be able to spend more time with their child during the holiday and would therefore be more likely to use the voucher. Indeed, the rural schools suggested that, as parents needed to have their own transportation to access some of the facilities, they would be more likely to make the trip.

Other comments indicated that there was a feeling that the voucher only catered for older children. This related to the issue of the time when activities were held at the leisure facilities. Examples indicated that some activities were only held during late evening sessions (badminton), therefore it was inappropriate to take younger children.

3.4 Project Management

All the schools visited had received support material as part of the initiative. Teachers believed that the appropriateness and quality of the material received was of benefit to the school. As previously stated, the reason for this opinion related to the fact that all had received support material relating to their greatest perceived needs:

- healthy eating;
- active/structured play;
- positive behaviour/social development.

However, a number of learning points emerged during the interviews, which primarily relate to the level and timing of information received regarding the initiative.

The interviews suggested that the Head Teachers were sent the Information Pack and order form in either early or late September 1997 (depending on whether they were in North or South Lanarkshire). However, the schools had already finalised their classroom activities for the year. Therefore, any support material requested was selected on the basis of ease of slotting it into what the school was already doing. As one teacher commented "ease of bolting it on to what we are already doing" Therefore, the initiative is not influencing schools in deciding to include key issues in the area of mental health, merely supporting existing activities within the classroom.

Consequently for the support material to have the greatest impact, schools need to be sent information at the end of term before the summer holiday or upon return after the break. In this way, teachers would be able to build the issues into classroom activities if suitable information was available regarding the options.

Another problem that emerged was that Head Teachers felt that the information received describing each option did not facilitate informed decision making when selecting their option. Whist the teachers appreciated the brevity of the Information Pack, they require more detailed information regarding the exact nature of the support material and possible examples of how it can be used in the classroom. Indeed, one teacher indicated that it would be useful if the Information Pack specifically linked the support material to the National Curriculum Guidelines, as this would improve the planning process.

The order form itself, proved to be slightly misleading as many Head Teachers were uncertain about the likelihood of receiving their first option. As a consequence, some selected all available options in the anticipation that they were then "bound to receive something". The confusion appears to have been caused by the opportunity to select a second option and the phrase " all topics are on a first come first served basis. We will endeavour to ensure you receive your first choice as far as possible" This seems to have created some uncertainty as to whether the school would receive any information or support material. Therefore the school was not counting on the support material when planning classroom activities.

Furthermore, impact on the planning process was further diminished as none of the Head Teachers were aware of the future likelihood that the initiative will be repeated. Consequently, they are not allocating any classroom time for Mental Health Week in 1998.

Some comments indicated that when support material was dispatched to the school, Head Teachers were not sure whether the pack had anything to do with the initiative. The confusion may have been caused by the fact that only a compliment slip was included in the Pack. However, the problem of poor branding is compounded by the fact that it is usually the teachers that use the material, not necessarily the person to which it is sent. Therefore, if the Head Teacher is not sure who the material has been sent from, by the time it reaches the classroom all identification / branding has been lost.

Another issue that emerged was in relation to the problem of information overload. One Head Teacher displayed a bookcase full of information packs. In his words "you'll never have enough time to read through all the material you receive". Therefore, it reinforces the need to look at the issue of branding material and supplying support material that closely meets the needs of the school.

4. Recommendations

In this section of the report, we build upon the available information to suggest a recommended course of action for the Health Promotion Department to consider.

1. We would strongly recommend that the initiative is repeated in future years, as there is a strong synergy with the school curriculum and teachers are supportive of the concept.

2. However, we believe that the Health Promotion Department should firstly consider at a strategic level the specific objectives of the initiative, to provide a more focussed approach.

3. The recent initiative provided something for all target groups' schools/ teachers/parents/children. However, the respondents believed that only the child related activities were of real value.

Therefore we would recommend that any future initiative focus support material on child related topics which support the school curriculum, so as to integrate Mental Health Week into planned classroom activities. The existing options that created most interest related to:

- healthy eating;
- exercise;
- positive behaviour.

Without question these are the areas that teachers currently believe are a priority in the children's development. By limiting the range of the available Options this will provide benefits to LHB with regard to budgeting for the initiative. This may then minimise schools' perception that they will not receive their selected support material.

4. We would recommend that the issue of the Admission Voucher scheme, in its current format, should not be repeated.

The distribution has to ensure that all parents receive the voucher and understand the nature of the event. Furthermore, the voucher should also try to encourage a change in behaviour. However, we believe the problems that exist with the distribution are insurmountable without incurring significantly greater costs. We also believe that even if the distribution was improved, this would still not change behaviour across the Socio Economic Groups that would benefit most from the vouchers. There are a number of external factors influencing behaviour, such as poor transportation links, the cost of public transportation and the overall cost of taking a family of more than one child to a leisure facility. Consequently, the voucher has a minimum impact on rural and low income families.

5. We would suggest that LHB consider the possibility of identifying key partner organisations that currently run similar initiatives within the primary school setting. During the course of the research we became aware of organisations such as Catering Direct and The Scottish Football Association which were running similar initiatives on Healthy Eating and Active Play. Therefore we believe that there is an opportunity to foster a collaborative approach which would ensure that a more co-ordinated message reaches the children.

6. With regard to the future project management of the initiative we strongly believe that LHB need to inform the schools of the longevity of the initiative and perhaps include an overview of the focus of the initiative in years to come. This will assist schools in the planning process when preparing curriculum activities. Therefore, any strategic review of the

initiative should perhaps consider possible themes that meet school curriculum requirements.

7. Specific information on the initiative needs to be issued to schools at the start of the summer term, at the latest. This will facilitate a possible influence on project work within the classroom, rather than providing support that may be in line with existing classroom projects.

8. Some thought should be given to the information pack that is issued to the schools. Whilst the information should be brief, it needs to detail the contents of the support material so the school knows exactly what resources will be available. Furthermore, where possible, specific linkages should be made to the National Curriculum Guidelines.

9. The style of future events should be given some thought as to the likely impact on changing behaviour and attitudes. For example, in relation to encouraging exercise it was felt that the children benefited from 'a before and after' fitness check. In this way, the children could recognise achievement which encouraged them to maintain their level of activity.

10. Also we would strongly suggest that, where possible, events should be based on the guest speaker approach. As discussed this type of event significantly improves the children's recall of the event and this in turn reinforces the message from the perceived 'specialist'.

27 Just Because I Like it Doesnt't Mean it has to Work: Personal Experience of an Antenatal Psychosocial Intervention Designed to Prevent Postnatal Depression

SANDRA L. WHEATLEY AND T. S. BRUGHA

Abstract

The antenatal psychosocial intervention to prevent postnatal depression 'Preparing for Parenthood' was evaluated in terms of the participants experiences of the classes in an additional study to compliment the findings of the core study with respect to the interventions immediate impact on their emotional well-being. All the women interviewed who attended the intervention considered it to be a positive experience. The immediate impact of the intervention was to increase, overall, the likelihood of depression. Therefore, the distinction between developing a 'pleasant' *and* an 'effective' health promotion intervention requires careful negotiation and longer term assessment.

Background

It makes sense that a demanding goal directed health promotion programme will benefit most those who find it credible and the psychological treatment evaluation literature provides some support for this (Hardy, *et al.* 1995). However, the benchmark of effectiveness in any new treatment commissioned by the National Health Service in England is evidence from randomised trials for which over £39 Million pounds has been allocated for the NHS's Health Technology Assessment programme (Anonymous, 1998). The present study provided an opportunity to explore these competing arguments, albeit on a modest scale, by introducing the essential research methodology of qualitative data collection and qualitative analysis.

The aim of the core study was to design and develop an antenatal intervention, Preparing for Parenthood, that reduces the four psychosocial risk factors of postnatal depression previously identified in this population from an earlier cohort study (N = 507 Brugha, *et al*. 1998). These were:

- the level of depression in pregnancy,
- an unplanned pregnancy,
- an unsupportive response to the pregnancy from the woman's partner and/or
- an unsupportive response to the pregnancy from the woman's mother.

The intervention draws on Parry's (1995) model of social support which emphasises cognitive and interpersonal processes. This intervention needed to address aspects of current cognition's. In particular, attitudes to pregnancy and motherhood, predictions of their future situation, and since prior depressive symptoms have been identified as a clear risk factor, these were also attended to. The format of the manual was based on an intervention manual that had been reported clearly, appeared to be easily replicable and of benefit to parents under stress (Kirkham, *et al*. 1988). Elements were added to increase clarity, to enhance the involvement of course leaders, and to increase the adherence of the participating women, drawing on work by Kirkham and Elliott (Elliott, *et al*. 1988). Personal problem solving, social support, information about PND, open sharing and cognitive aspects were the 5 central components. The core study investigated the intervention's ability to reduce and/or prevent postnatal depression utilising the quantitative design of an RCT.

A separate set of intervention classes was organised to investigate how the women perceived and experienced the intervention using qualitative methods. This separation ensured that the randomised control trial design, which used purely quantitative methods, was not compromised. The procedures for the qualitative study were otherwise identical to the core trial study so that comparisons could confidently be made. This paper reports findings from the additional qualitative study.

Procedure

Screening

Women in their first pregnancy, due to have their baby in February, March, or April 1998, and attending their first antenatal clinic were screened, using the 12 item General Health Questionnaire identified in work by Surtees and Miller (1990), including all of the 6 depression items (GHQ-Depression). These were embedded in a short self completion questionnaire called 'Pregnancy & You', which focuses on the key support deficits identified in the earlier prospective cohort research. Participation required the written informed consent of each woman according to a protocol agreed by the Leicestershire Research Ethics Committee.

As in a previous cohort study in the same antenatal clinic (Brugha, *et al.* 1998) 15-20% were predicted to be identified as at high risk, consenting and eligible for inclusion. Therefore, screening was estimated to need to be carried out on up to 100 women so that 20 women would scored positive (antenatal GHQ-Depression greater than or equal to one). Of these 20 women it was anticipated that between two thirds and a half would want to take part in the intervention. This would mean a group size of between 10 and 15 women for the intervention classes.

Intervention

The intervention, 'Preparing for Parenthood' consisted of 6 antenatal classes, preceded by an initial introductory meeting with the participant, and followed later by a postnatal reunion class when the babies were about 8 weeks old. The intervention was fully documented in a training and operational manual that included checklists and feedback forms for completion by course participants and by course leaders and will be reported in more detail elsewhere in 1999.

The initial meetings lasted about half an hour and were an opportunity for the women to come and meet their course leaders who answered any questions about the intervention and helped with problems they may anticipate having getting to the classes.

The following themes were the focus of at least one group:

- being aware of and acknowledging problems,
- facts about emotional problems and postnatal depression,
- support and effective support seeking,
- and problem solving with the help of others.

At these groups, difficulties with partners and other family members and how they appear to fall short of expectation could be discussed. Women were encouraged to support each other and to seek and obtain practical advice and assistance in relation to any other problems and to make use of their midwifery team as a continuing source of support. Based on the earlier cohort, a strong focus was placed on the woman's future material circumstances after child birth including her housing, income sources, and dependency on others.

A meeting open to the partner or significant other, with an educational focus, also took place for which the 2 group leaders were joined by an additional male nurse who worked with the participants male partners. Cognitive behavioural techniques were used in both settings, where appropriate, in order to restructure the women's perceptions of potentially available support from key others. All of the classes were antenatal and were scheduled not to clash with parentcraft classes, which tend to be held later and focus on obstetric care and infant care.

A final 'reunion' class took place approximately two to three months after childbirth, at which the women were encouraged to renew their friendships and explore ways of continuing to obtain the support they need before any problems become insurmountable.

The women's emotional well-being was assessed using the brief reliable and valid self-completion measure, the Edinburgh Postnatal Depression Scale (EPDS) (Cox, et al. 1997), at the initial meeting and at the sixth and final session.

The intervention was carried out following exactly the same procedures in the additional qualitative study as for the core trial study and was run by course leaders drawn from the same pool. The only difference was that this particular set of intervention sessions were video-taped for a parallel study exploring the adherence of course leaders to the intervention package and the interactions amongst the women group members with each other and the course leaders. The results of this adherence study will not be reported here.

Postnatal Interview

All women who either attended the intervention (compliant), did not attend the intervention (non-compliant), or who declined the invitation to attend the intervention (refusers) were contacted by post between one and two months postnatally. The letter explained that regardless of whether or not they had managed to come along to the classes, their experiences of the research project were of value to us and would help us to monitor and improve our research methods. The letter also informed them that the interview would be audiotaped for the use of the research team only.

The interview consisted of 9 questions constructed to explore fully the core areas of interest within this study. The questionnaire was designed to facilitate the method of qualitative analysis to be used i.e. Grounded theory.

Results

Emotional Well-being of Sample to be Interviewed

The table below shows the GHQ-D and EPDS scores of the women in the sample over the study period (where available i.e. if they came to that session, N/A = non-attendance of that session). From the table it can be seen that the participant women's emotional well-being fluctuated over the period of their pregnancy's with the majority of women scoring below the cut-point of 13 on the EPDS which serves as an indicator of vulnerability to postnatal depression.

Table 1 Emotional well-being of the qualitative study sample

Name	Sub-sample	Screening GHQ-D	Initial Meeting EPDS	Session 6 EPDS
Emma	Compliant	2	10	17
Helen	Compliant	2	8	6
Claire	Compliant	1	3	9
Ameena	Compliant	1	6	11
Samantha	Non-compliant	1	9	N/A
Tanya	Non-compliant	2	9	N/A
Sarah	Non-compliant	1	16	N/A
Michelle	Non-compliant **	1	N/A	N/A
Rachel	Non-compliant	1	N/A	N/A
Pritty	Non-compliant **	2	N/A	N/A
Catherine	Refuser **	2	N/A	N/A
Sadie	Refuser	1	N/A	N/A

Main Themes Identified from the Qualitative Analysis

As with all qualitative analysis the influence of the interviewers perspective will have had an impact upon the perspectives of the responses gained from

271

the interviewees. However, one interviewer completed all of the interviews and attempted to maintain the same open frame of mind throughout the nine interviews completed. Only complete interviews were included in the analysis to identify the main themes of the sample of interviews by the grounded theory technique. The interviews were analysed as an entire sample rather than as three discreet sub-groups. This was done primarily because it was believed that as few boundaries as possible should be imposed on the data to maximise the identification of themes running through the interviews. The interviewers speech is shown in italics and the participants responses as normal text.

The themes identified relevant to this paper can be separated into two categories. Firstly, that of PND - what the women know, what they want to know or did not want to know, and whether they thought the classes would help. Secondly, the women's perception of the intervention and its relevance to their everyday lives.

Individual assessment of need for information about postnatal depression
The majority of women knew very little if anything at all about PND; there was no real difference between the three engagement sub-samples of compliant, non-compliant and refuser.

> *So you had heard about postnatal depression, and you had a bit of experience with your sister, so did you know kind of what symptoms to look for or?*
> No.
> *You'd just kind of heard of the name?*
> That's right.
> (Emma, compliant, responses 63 - 64)

> *What had you heard about postnatal depression, before I spoke to you in the antenatal clinic? ... Had you heard of it?*
> Yes I had heard of it. But I didn't know that much really, I knew what to look out for in myself, but I didn't have much information. Mostly from magazines and that.
> (Tanya, non-compliant, response 31)

Many women were aware of this knowledge gap. Their perception of their need for information about PND seems to have been a preoccupation with most of them at some point in their pregnancy, whether they went on to seek or avoid information. A dichotomy of the women's perceptions of what

272

their lack of knowledge would mean to them became clearly apparent. The two concepts with their associated themes are described below. Unfortunately, the amount of illustrative quotes would be too grand to accommodate in this section.

1. Lack of knowledge = protective factor: Generally, these women avoid information, see their behaviour as not tempting fate, hope it won't happen, also, they didn't give the impression of having control of their emotions and did not seem to want the responsibility of the potential consequences of having control of their emotions.
2. Lack of knowledge = vulnerability factor: Generally, these women felt exposed, they felt they were at risk of losing control of their emotions and feared not having control, they actively sought support from significant others and from individuals with previous experience of the situation they were currently experiencing, specifically they wanted facts and strategies for coping with every eventuality.

The quotes below illustrate this as some women sought information about postnatal depression, however, the majority of the women interviewed admitted to avoiding information about postnatal depression.

The thought of postnatal depression, that you could be that one woman in ten, how did that make you feel?
I didn't think it was too unrealistic to be honest, because of how I felt at the time. But, I obviously wanted to avoid it.
Yes.
So, I wanted to do something about it. It wasn't there at that stage, but I thought it was a possibility if I carried on thinking the way I was thinking. Not being able to shift it or see things in a different light. So I had to do something about it.
(Helen, compliant, responses 52 - 53)

So why did you want to know about postnatal depression ?
Errmm, well, basically, so that I didn't get it, you know…
And did you think about it, that you might get it?
Errmm, I didn't think I was going to get it. No,no. I just wanted to read about …
(Claire, compliant, responses 15 - 16)

I try to never let it cross me mind really cos I always thought well I want this baby so surely I won't get it, so I never really thought about

What, you tried not to think about it?
Yeah, I think that was it.
So you went out of your way not to.
Yeah I think that was, I say like I never asked about it so .. You don't want it to happen do you so you think well you'll just forget about it, I think that's what I did really.
(Samantha, non-compliant, responses 64 - 68)

Did you find out anything more about postnatal depression, from you doctor or your midwife?
Well no not really. I just didn't want to know. I think I thought if I didn't know about it, it wouldn't happen [laughs].
That it would go away?
Yeah, yeah [little laugh again] Silly really.
(Tanya, non-compliant, responses 35 - 36)

The only woman to place no value on the classes was in fact the refuser. However, later in the interview she appeared to have changed her mind. She went on to say what she felt she had missed out on and what she wished she had been told about pregnancy and how she would feel when she had her baby. These overlapped with the main contents of the intervention quite considerably. The contents of the classes either weren't communicated adequately at the initial contact in the antenatal clinic with the screening questionnaire or simply were not salient to this woman at that time.

You weren't too sure. Why weren't you too sure ?
I think, you feel like a bit strange walking into a room full of people who know each other , where you don't , I don't think it would have made any difference.
So... You don't think it would have made any difference at all?
No.
So, learning about coping, support, the birth, things like that...?
No.
(Sadie, refuser, responses 19-21)

Ok.....If you could turn the clock back to when I saw you in the antenatal clinic, would your decision to attend or not attend our classes {Preparing for parenthood} be different now? Would you decide you didn't want to go?
I would go. I wish I could turn the clock back. Yeah.
Oh, and why's that?

Yeah learn sort of more about, know what to, and what to do. I weren't sure what I was doing, being pregnant was all about.
(Sadie, refuser, responses 100-102)

Women felt that attending the classes was a positive experience Whether the women came to one session or six sessions they all enjoyed the classes and said that they would make the same decision to come to these classes again when (if!) they had their second child.

I am glad I attended I did get quite a lot out of it. it was mainly to do with support. A lot of the meetings was about making friends, I've got a busy life, now if I feel I'm not good at anything we can just ring each other. *So that relaxed you, you feel like you got something out of it?* Yeah, friendship.
......
Initially, I thought oh no how boring, but then as it progressed it got a lot more interesting and I must admit it did help, the classes did help me in terms of asking for support.
......
If you could turn the clock back to when I saw you when you were pregnant, would your decision to do the PFP classes be different now? I would definitely still have done the classes, definitely, oh yes.
(Ameena, compliant, responses 19 - 21, 44 & 140)

Those women that did not make it to all the sessions of the intervention wished that they had been able to come along - whatever the main obstacle was to them not attending more sessions (if they had attended any).

I mean I wish I hadn't missed the others, you know what I mean, to carry on really but just what with getting there as well as my bleeding...., so like, you know, I was upset that I missed quite a few sessions.
(Samantha, non-compliant, response 88)

Most of the women who had attended the intervention in some part found that what they had learnt was useful and could be applied to their everyday life. They mentioned that they had, amongst other aspects; gained confidence, developed the ability to generate different perspectives on problems, and felt that they were now able to be tactful, successful and remain in control when asking for and turning down support.

275

So almost being allowed to ask them was, that it was OK to ask, that its not a weakness
Yes
Other people do it, its fairly simple. And before?
Usually I'm not like that . I just struggle through myself, get on with it .... so yes I do ask for help now!
(Ameena, compliant, responses 46 - 51)

Did you find that you were using the information you'd been given in the classes?
Errm ..A bit yeah, especially the SODAS system {problem solving}, I felt I should be stopping and thinking you know, when I did try and cope I was sort of trying to stop and, you know, work my way through it
Do you still do it now or ?
Not so much, but I mean I know I suppose its made me think a bit more, how I feel in the situation rather than just jumping straight forward [laughs]
So you're sort of evaluating different things that you could do.
Yeah, what sort of options that I've got to deal with the problem.
(Sarah, non-compliant, responses 62 - 64)

Yeah, that was fine, it was good, learning things, you know social support, turning it down, asking for help...
Yeah,
I think my problem is, my mum was very fussy when I was pregnant, she kept saying oh let me do this for you. I didn't want her to. It's not because I didn't want to ask for help, I knew I could do it, and she made me feel that I couldn't do it.
Yeah,
Like she'd say oh do you want me call round and do some ironing or do you want me to work for you tonight, and I'd say 'no I'm OK', and she couldn't understand why, why I'd end up snapping at her. I'd say to her, look , one day you know I am going to need your help, but at the moment I don't need it, and she couldn't understand. She'd say oh I'm not going to ask if you want my help anymore, but she did, you know. [laughs]
(Claire, compliant, responses 49 - 51)

Discussion

Although women found the intervention reassuring, interesting, beneficial, relevant, and thought provoking; the results of the randomised trial, reported elsewhere, clearly revealed that it did not improve their emotional well-being in the longer term beyond. Whilst attention should be paid to the experiences of participants, to ascertain whether these experiences have had a significant impact on their emotional well-being, such information should be cautiously interpreted. Even the use of quantitative outcome measures within a period of time with a series of clients can lead to misleading conclusions about the effectiveness and the quality of care (Brugha & Lindsay, 1996).

Therefore the implications from this study are by no means uncomplicated. It can be confidently concluded that this is an intervention that is thoroughly acceptable to first-time mothers identified as at heightened risk of postnatal depression. Clarifying the distinction between 'effective' health promotion and 'pleasant' health promotion would appear to be an issue not to be ignored by researchers, health promotion workers or policy makers.

References

Brugha, T.S., & Lindsay, F. (1996) 'Quality of mental health service care: the forgotten pathway from process to outcome', *Social Psychiatry and Psychiatric Epidemiology* 31, pp. 89-98.

Brugha, T.S., Sharp, H.M., Cooper, S.A., Weisender, C., Britto, D., Shinkwin, R., Sherrif, T., & Kirwan, P.H. (1998) 'The Leicester 500 project. Social support and the development of postnatal depressive symptoms, a prospective cohort survey', *Psychological Medicine* 28, pp. 63-79.

Cox, J.L., Holden, J.M, & Sagovsky, R. (1987) 'Detection of postnatal depression. Development of the 10 item Edinburgh Postnatal Depression Scale', *British Journal of Psychiatry* 150, pp.782-786.

Elliott, S.A., Sanjack, M., & Leverton, T.J. (1988) 'Parents groups in pregnancy. A preventative intervention for postnatal depression?', in B.H. Gottlieb (ed), *Marshalling social support* (pp. 87-110), Sage, Beverly Hills.

Hardy, G.E., Barkham, M., Shapiro, D.A., Reynolds, S., Rees, A., & Stiles, W.B. (1995). 'Credibility and outcome of cognitive-behavioural and psychodynamic-interpersonal psychotherapy', *British Journal of Clinical Psychology* 34, pp. 555-569.

Kirkham, M.A., Norelius, L., Meltzer, N.J. Schilling, R.F., & Schinke, S.P., *(1988) Reducing stress in mothers of children with special needs*, University of Washington Press.

NHS Executive (1998) *The Annual Report of the NHS Health Technology Assessment Programme 1998*, NHS Executive.

Parry, G. (1995) 'Social support processes and cognitive therapy' in T.S.Brugha (ed), *Social support and psychiatric disorder: research findings and guidelines for clinical practice.* (pp.279-294), Cambridge University Press, Cambridge.

Surtees, P.G., & Miller, P.M. (1990) 'The interval General Health Questionnaire', *British Journal of Psychiatry* 157, pp.686-693.

Acknowledgements

This study was supported by a grant from the NHS R&D National Mental Health Programme, with additional support from the Leicestershire Mental Health NHS Trust R&D Programme and from the Section of Social Psychiatry, Department of Psychiatry, University of Leicester.

For Product Safety Concerns and Information please contact our EU
representative GPSR@taylorandfrancis.com
Taylor & Francis Verlag GmbH, Kaufingerstraße 24, 80331 München, Germany